Communication Skills for Nursing Practic

First edition 2006
Second edition 2013
Published by
PALGRAVE MACMILLAN

Palgrave Macmillan in the UK is an imprint of Macmillan Publishers Limited, registered in England, company number 785998, of Houndmills, Basingstoke, Hampshire RG21 6XS.

Palgrave Macmillan in the US is a division of St Martin's Press LLC, 175 Fifth Avenue, New York, NY 10010.

Palgrave Macmillan is the global academic imprint of the above companies and has companies and representatives throughout the world.

Palgrave® and Macmillan® are registered trademarks in the United States, the United Kingdom, Europe and other countries

ISBN: 978–0–230–36920–7 paperback

This book is printed on paper suitable for recycling and made from fully managed and sustained forest sources. Logging, pulping and manufacturing processes are expected to conform to the environmental regulations of the country of origin.

A catalogue record for this book is available from the British Library.

A catalog record for this book is available from the Library of Congress.

Typeset by Cambrian Typesetters, Camberley, Surrey

Communication Skills for Nursing Practice

2nd Edition

Catherine McCabe
and
Fiona Timmins

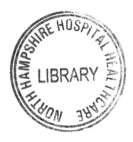

palgrave
macmillan

Contents

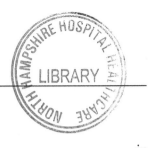

List of Figures and Tables

Figures

Tables

Acknowledgements

We would like to thank our colleagues in the School of Nursing and Midwifery, University of Dublin, Trinity College Dublin, for their support and encouragement throughout the preparation of the 2nd edition of this textbook. We are also grateful to the staff at Palgrave Macmillan for their invaluable support. Finally we are indebted to the late Jo Campling for her contribution towards both the conception and completion of this book.

The authors and publishers wish to thank: Elsevier Ltd for permission to reproduce Fig 1.1 Circular Transactional Model of Communication, originally published in *Interpersonal Relationships: Professional Communication Skills for Nurses 6th edition*, by Arnold, E.C. & Underman Bogg, K., (Fig 2.1, pg 14) © Elsevier 2011, Fig 2.1 The Model of Living and Fig 2.2 Individualizing nursing as a dynamic process using the Roper-Logan-Tierney Model of Nursing, both originally published in *The Roper Logan Tierney Model of Nursing Based on Activities of Living,* by Roper N. Logan and Tierney, A.J, (pg 14 Fig 2.1 and pg 142 Fig 3.8 respectively) © Elsevier 2001, Fig 2.4 A Diagramatic Representation of Peplau's Developmental Model, originally published in Pearson, *Nursing Models for Practice,* 3rd edition, by Pearson et al, Butterworth Heinemann © 2000, 2005, and Fig 8.1 Assertive Rights, originally published in Teaching Assertiveness to Undergraduate Nursing Students, by McCabe C., and Timmins, F. in *Nurses Education in Practice,* 3:1 pp30–42 © Elsevier 2003; John Wiley and Sons for permission to reproduce Fig 1.2 Model of Communication, originally published in Beyond Empathy by Morse et al in *Journal of Advanced Nursing* (pp809–821) © 2006; Springer Publishing Company Inc for permission to reproduce Fig 2.3 Overlapping Phases in Nurse–Patient Relationships originally published in *Interpersonal relations in nursing: a conceptual frame of reference for psychodynamic nursing* by Peplau, H © 1991; Nursing and Midwifery Council (NMC) for permission to reproduce selected competencies in Table 5.2 Field competencies related to the domain of communication and interpersonal skills for adult nurses, originally from *Field Competencies for Adult Nurses* © NMC 2010 and The McGraw-Hill Companies, Inc for Fig 10.1 The Johari Window, originally published in *Group Process: an Introduction to Group Dynamics, 3rd edition* by Luft, J. © McGraw-Hill Companies 1984.

PART I

The Theoretical Foundations of Communication in Nursing

1 Communication Theory

Introduction

The basis for communication lies in sharing a common existence with others but with each as a unique individual within the mix of human life. This represents the phenomenological view of communication as dialogue between self and others and although it should be considered in the context of other theories presented in this text book it provides a sound basis for the beginning of our discussion of communication (Craig 2001). Communication is something that we all do whether we want to or not, even if we hide ourselves away and cannot be seen, we are still communicating that we are unhappy or do not wish to see other people. We cannot prevent ourselves from communicating, even if we try not to speak to someone, our bodies will betray us and send a message to the other person. So we are all compelled to communicate at some level by using language and our bodies. However, communication does not always seem to work effectively. Why is this? Why do we walk away from encounters feeling angry, humiliated, frustrated and thinking to ourselves, 'if only I had said...'. On the other hand why do we walk away from situations leaving others feeling like this? Indeed, how often are we actually aware that our communication has possibly engendered negative feelings in others?

The basis for communication lies in our common existence with others in a shared world that may be constituted differently in experience.

Exercise

To what extent are you aware of the impact of your communication behaviours on others? You may write down your thoughts on this before proceeding with the chapter.

Exercise

'What is Communication'? Try to write down the first ideas that come into your head and keep them close by, as you will need to refer back to them as you read on.

It could be argued that communication is not actually communication unless it is intentional. When communicating, you need to consider and be aware of the effect your facial expression and tone has on another person. Your behaviour whether verbal or non-verbal, will influence how another person communicates with you because of the message that your tone and body language sends out. For example, if you are distracted and irritable because you have received a letter telling you that you have been caught speeding in your car and will have to pay a fine and get points on your licence, and this is evident in your facial expression and tone when you are speaking to a work colleague or patient about an unrelated matter, then it affects the interaction.

This book is concerned with interpersonal communication in nursing, regardless of the medium through which it takes place. The emphasis is on the verbal and/or non-verbal language required to deliver the message in a manner that is patient-centred, respectful, genuine and therapeutic. This requires a level of awareness, not just of the specific nature and purpose of the message but most importantly it requires knowledge of one's self. Communication is about interacting with people and therefore is at the core of nursing. For nursing care to be effective and therapeutic, the communication skills used by nurses need to be positive and patient-centred. This requires a continuing awareness by nurses as individuals of their contribution to interactions that they have not just with patients but also with relatives, friends, other healthcare professionals and healthcare staff. Nurses spend more time with patients than any other healthcare professional and coordinate their care by communicating closely with other professionals. Without attempting to define all aspects of the nurse's role, communication is without doubt an integral part of the nurse's role. The collaborative skills required to do this well and effectively are discussed in Chapter 7.

Defining communication

This chapter explores communication as a concept; first, by reviewing non-nursing communication models frequently referred to when we think or learn about communication. Second, in order to consider communication in a context that we believe is unique to nursing, models of communication specific to nursing are also reviewed. However, before that let us look at various definitions of communication:

'A process in which the individual implements a set of goal-directed inter-related, situationally appropriate social behaviours, which are learned and controlled' (Hargie 2006: 13).

'Human communication consists of the sending and receiving of verbal and nonverbal messages between two or more people' (DeVito 2011). DeVito adds the comment to this definition that although this appears to be a simple process it is quite complex in reality.

'Communication involves the reciprocal process in which messages are sent and received between two or more people' (Balzer-Riley 2011: 6).

'A useful way of thinking about interpersonal communication is as a series of messages – information – which you send out to other people and messages which you received from them, through seeing, hearing or touching one another' (Petrie 1997: 6).

'Communication is a universal function of man that is not tied to any particular place, time or context' (Ruesch 1961: 30–1).

The diversity of these definitions in terms of their broadness or even vagueness highlights the complexity of the concept of communication and therefore, the difficulty in producing a comprehensive model and definition of communication that truly reflects its essence. In their definitions, of communication, Hargie (2011), Balzer-Riley (2011), Petrie (1997) and Hayes (1991) all use terms such as 'interpersonal communication' and 'interpersonal skills' interchangeably and are based on the fundamental belief that communication is an interpersonal process. Ruesch (1961) did not concur with this view. His definition described communication as a function, which implied that it is always purposeful. However, none of these definitions or models provides possible explanations as to why some communication is positive and some is not. Consider the following interaction.

> Smiling and in a friendly tone, a nurse asks her nursing colleague, 'Are you free to check the medication with me now'? Her colleague is reading some notes and she looks and sounds irritated when she replies, 'Yes, ok but it will have to be quick; the new admission will be here in fifteen minutes'. The first nurse seems confused by this reaction and says 'If you are busy I will ask someone else'. Her colleague immediately says 'No, no, I'm sorry if I seem irritable, it's just that I was looking at the duty roster and I am working on my birthday.'

This type of interaction is quite a common between colleagues or friends and is an example of both intrapersonal and interpersonal communication. The colleague probably did look irritated but this was due to her own private thoughts in relation to having to work on her birthday and her face registered these inner feelings. However, the first nurse perceived the irritated expression as being directed at them. The problem is that often an individual's intrapersonal communication is evident in their facial expression and a message is sent to the outside and is observed and interpreted by other people but this message is not or was never intended to be a message to another person. This is an example of unconscious communication that can have a negative effect on an interaction. The nurses communicated well in this example and nobody was left feeling negative about the interaction but often such interactions can cause friction and bad feeling among colleagues. Of course, the opposite is also possible, that is, communication that is successful and has a positive outcome can also be the result of communication that is unconscious.

Concepts of communication

Depending on the model structure and underpinning concept, communication can be regarded as both simple and a complex process. The Linear Model of Communication (Miller and Nicholson, 1976) may be considered as an illustration of simple communication. This is illustrated as follows:

Sender → Message → Receiver

Berlo (1960) and Miller and Nicholson (1976) described communication as a simple activity in which a sender transmits a message to a receiver in order to bring about a desired response. Communication is said to occur in one direction only. The sender is responsible for not only the accuracy of the content but also the tone of the message. The message contains verbal and/or non-verbal information that will be interpreted by the receiver. The sender of the message will know that the receiver has interpreted the message accurately through feedback.

However, based on this model, for communication to be effective it is assumed that sender is very clear about the purpose of the message and what it is supposed to achieve and has also carefully considered the recipient when formulating the message. It is also assumed that, in this model, the recipient is an open-minded and willing participant in the interaction. These assumptions do not take into account other factors (intrinsic and extrinsic factors) that can influence the communication process. Intrinsic factors apply to both the sender and receiver and refer to personal and professional aspects of a person that may affect communication. Examples of these are values, beliefs, culture, goals, role and knowledge/education in relation to the topic of communication. Extrinsic factors relate to the immediate physical environment and the communication medium being used. DeVito (2011) described these factors as 'noise' that could distort the message being transmitted and distort the perception of the receiver, such that the message is interpreted differently to the original meaning intended by the sender. DeVito (2000) described four types of noise:

physical noise (external to the speaker, e.g., loud music or voices in the background);
physiological noise (physical impairments that influence perception by the receiver);
psychological noise (perceptions of sender/receiver being influenced by individual beliefs, values, biases, goals); and
semantic noise (words have different meanings in different contexts).

The Linear Model of Communication is, therefore, limited and perhaps is most useful for identifying the basic components of simple communication, rather than for illustrating the complexities of communication between humans.

The Circular Transactional Model of Communication, based on the work of Bateson (1979) takes a broader view of the communication process (Figure 1.1). Communication comprises similar components as the linear model but the concept of communication is further developed by the indication that all

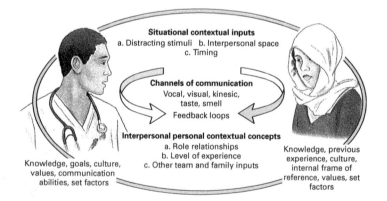

Figure 1.1 Picture of circular transactional model of communication

Source: Arnold E.C. and Underman Boggs, K. (2011) *Interpersonal relationships–Professional communication skills for nurses*. 6th Edition. Saunders, St Louis. Reproduced with kind permission from Elsevier Ltd

communication is interpersonal, therefore, it takes place within the context of a relationship. This model acknowledges the key role that intrinsic and extrinsic factors outlined above or 'noise' play in the communication process but it also included the concepts of 'feedback' and 'validation' as fundamental for the development and continuation of successful or effective communication.

Both of these concepts will be discussed in Chapter 3 in relation to therapeutic communication. The transactional nature of this model lies in its recognition of communication as a reciprocal process in which communication is simultaneous and shared between people as 'communicators' rather than a 'sender' and 'receiver'. The cyclical aspect of this model acknowledges that communication is not linear or one-way but is instead an ongoing dynamic process that is inherently complex.

Harms (2007) describes a multidimensional approach to communication that comprises of seven key themes:

1. An individual's inner world is multidimensional and unique.
2. An individual's outer world that influences their inner world to shape their daily life experiences.
3. Time is multidimensional comprising biological, biographical, historical/social, cyclical and future elements that influence behaviour and experience.
4. Experience is multidimensional and unique to individuals.
5. Adaptation is multidimensional and shapes individual or group responses to adversity thus allowing others to comment on/predict behaviour, risk, vulnerability and resilience.
6. Theorizing human development and adaptation should be multidimensional in order to provided human service responses that are appropriate and effective.
7. Human service responses must be multidimensional

This is an interesting model because it shows the origin of unique individual communication behaviour in the experiences of everyday life and the importance of considering the multidimensional approach when working with people and developing appropriate services (Harms 2007).

Hargie's (2011) model of communication 'A Skills Model of Interpersonal Communication' contains many of the elements illustrated in the circular transaction model of communication and Harms' (2007) model but in contrast it presents these elements as skills, suggesting that effective or successful interpersonal communication is purposeful and focused. These skills are identified as follows:

- person–situation context;
- goal;
- mediating processes;
- response;
- feedback; and
- perception.

The person–situation context refers to the individual or unique aspects of a person that contributes to an interaction. These aspects include the person's values, beliefs, culture knowledge, skills, personality, age, gender, self-concept and self-efficacy (self-belief in one's ability to succeed) and may influence their approach and style of response during an inter-action. The situation itself in terms of not just the physical setting but also the parameters (roles and rules) will also directly impact how people behave and respond during an interaction.

The goal of the individuals involved in the interaction may be the same or it may differ to a greater or lesser degree. The achievement of the goal influences each participant's behaviour and persistence. Success also depends on whether the goals are implicit or explicit, how important they are, whether they are task or relationship related, how compatible the goals of the people are and whether they are primary or secondary goals.

Mediating processes refer to a combination of cognitive and affective processes that help the participants in the interaction to work through the encounter by identifying goals and acknowledging and responding to events. Cognitive processes are concerned with how individuals have a very personal way of using their knowledge and beliefs when thinking about things and this directly impacts on how they solve problems, make judgments or perceive situations generally. The affective process is based on an individual's value system and the way in which it influences our attitude towards our actions and interactions with others. A crucial aspect of mediating processes is that a tentative or flexible outcome (strategy or plan for achieving a goal) is reached.

The 'response' aspect of the skills model relates to the implementation of the agreed strategy or plan. Responses incorporate the use of verbal and non-verbal communication, which along with environmental and organizational factors can influence the smooth or bumpy implementation of the strategy or plan.

Feedback is described by Hargie (2011) as an integral ingredient in the communication process because it lets everyone in the interaction know that the message has been received and also lets the sender know how those who received it have interpreted it. Feedback is evident from both verbal and non-verbal responses equally and clarifies whether interpretation or understanding of the message is mutual or shared. This allows the communication to continue and strategies and plans to be refined and implemented.

Perception refers to the way we perceive others and the context in which an interaction takes place is the primary influence on what happens in the interaction and also what the outcome of the interaction is. In order to predict how an interaction will proceed and its outcome, we need to be aware of and monitor ourselves in terms of our performance and contribution to the interaction and that failure to do this may result in regular experiences of ineffective communication or unwanted outcomes from interactions (Hargie 2011).

It is difficult to define communication and looking at the models presented it is clear to see why. The linear model represents communication as one directional and does not recognize the influence of the individual or the environment in the communication process and the complexities therein. The circular transactional model is broader in that it recognizes the influence that the individual and the context have on the communication process and the importance of feedback and validation in allowing the interaction to be interpreted and expected outcome to be agreed. The 'Skills Model of Interpersonal Communication' is based on similar components but includes key ingredients such as the goal of the interaction, individual perceptions, and the mediating processes that play a fundamental role in the development and outcome of an interaction. This model introduces the notion that communication requires certain behavioural skills in order to be successful for all those involved in the interaction. It can certainly be argued now that communication is not a simple process in any interaction or situation and to regard it as such would require that the dynamic individual and contextual nature of communication be ignored or underestimated.

Mindful of this and in view of the models of communication reviewed we propose that communication is best described as a complex, unconscious or deliberate process that influences the development of interpersonal or professional relationships and outcomes of interactions, regardless of the context.

Exercise

Earlier in this chapter you were asked to consider what you think communication is and write it down. Now having read about some communication models and definitions have a look at what you have written and decide whether you want to make any adjustments. When you are happy with this, answer these questions;

● What is communication in nursing?
● Is it different to communication in the other healthcare professionals?
● Again, write down the thoughts that come into your head and keep them, as you will need to refer to them again when you have finished this chapter and others in this book.

Models of communication in nursing

We regard communication in nursing as different to communication in other healthcare professions. It is unique, not because of the communication skills required as any professional working with the public needs to have effective communications skills, but rather because of the focus and emphasis of communication in the professional practice of nursing. Nurses are key members of healthcare services. They spend more time with patients than perhaps any other health-care professional. The focus of this time is often on coordinating, explaining and delivering patient care using therapeutic communication. The emphasis of this time (or should be) is facilitating individual patients needs. It is widely recognized that communication is practically unavoidable and is to do with people interacting and developing relationships and working and living together. Therefore, it follows that as nursing is about helping people, the communication of information and feelings between the nurse and the patient and the nurse and other healthcare professionals is an integral part of how nurses do their job. Authors such as Peplau (1988), Sheppard (1993), Fosbinder (1994), Wilkinson (1999), Attree (2001) and Thorsteinsson (2002) support this view and also suggest that the development of a positive nurse–patient relationship is essential for the delivery of high-quality nursing care.

Previously in this chapter we looked at three models of communication. It became evident that the linear model, which depicts one-way communication, is limited in its application and not congruent with the multidimensional nature of communication in nursing. The circular transactional model and the skills model of interpersonal communication are certainly more useful in explaining the processes and components of interpersonal communication required in nursing.

There are very few models of communication that relate to specifically to nursing, however, authors such as Fosbinder (1994) and Morse et al.(1992) and Morse et al.(1997) have made significant contributions to this aspect of nursing. In her study, Fosbinder (1994) asked patients to describe what happened when the nurse was taking care of them. The inter-personal competence of the nurse was the primary concern of the patients and four interpersonal processes emerged from their descriptions:

- Translating – the key components of this include information giving, explaining and instructing.
- Getting to know you relates to being friendly, using humour in interactions and personal sharing.
- Establishing trust – this relates to the confidence that patients have in the nurse's professional competence and demeanour. It requires that nurses anticipate patient need, follow through and appear to enjoy the job.
- Going the 'extra mile' relates to being a friend and doing more for the patient than is required. This is not something that patients expect from every nurse but it is described as a special, less formal relationship between a nurse and patient.

As you can see the main focus of these four processes is interpersonal competence and communication and if you consider the components of each of these processes, the communication skills required are not highly specialized, most of us either use them already or could achieve them without even realizing it. What makes this model so important and relevant is that its content is derived directly from patients and therefore provides key information to nurses about how patients want them to communicate.

Morse et al.(1992) developed a model of communication that focused on the emotional engagement of the nurse with the patient (Figure 1.2). The model is based on two key characteristics. The first is whether the nurse is patient-focused or nurse-focused and the second is whether the communication is spontaneous (first-level) or learned (second-level). The patient-focused, first-level communication is emotionally driven and culturally conditioned and is therefore often an unconscious response. This type of communication includes responses such as pity, sympathy, consolation, compassion, commiseration and reflexive reassurance, which we would often regard as normal every day communication but is often undervalued and regarded as superficial (Morse et al.1992, McQueen, 2000). Sympathy, for example, which Morse et al. (1992: 812) defined as 'an expression of the caregiver's own sorrow at another's plight' can make patients feel understood and comforted because the nurse has recognized how unwell they may be

FOCUS

		Sufferer-focused (patient)		Self-focused (professional)	
		CHARACTERISTIC	RESPONSE	RESPONSE	CHARACTERISTIC
First-level		Engaged (with sufferer's emotion) Genuine Reflexive	Pity Sympathy Consolation Commiseration Compassion Reflexive reassurance	Guarding Shielding/steeling/ bracing Dehumanizing Withdrawing Distancing Labelling Denying	Anti-engaged (against embodiment; protective)

Second-level		Pseudo-engaged
		
		Learned
		Professional
			Sharing self
			Humour
			Reassurance
			(informing)
			Therapeutic
			  empathy
			Confronting
			Comforting
			(learned)
				Rote behaviours
				  'professional style'
				Legitimizing/
				justifying
				Pity
				  (false/
				  professional)
				Stranger
				Reassurance (false)
					A-engaged
					
					(embodiment
					absent or removed)

Figure 1.2   A model of communication

Source: Morse, J.M., De Luca Havens, G.A., & Wilson, S. The comforting inter-action: Developing a model of nurse–patient relationship, *Scholarly Inquiry for Nursing Practice*, © 2006 John Wiley and Son Ltd. Reproduced with kind permission from John Wiley and Sons

feeling. This narrative from a study on nurse-patient communi-cation by McCabe (2004: 45) illustrates this point,

> I liked them (nurses) all, but there was one little girl, she was slightly different – sympathetic I would say. I think the patient deserves sympathy when they are hospitalized, their complaint may not warrant sympathy but they're away from their own environment (Sophie).

Patient-focused, second-level (learned) communication includes responses such as sharing self, confronting, comfort-ing, humour and informative reassurance. These responses may be difficult for some nurses at undergraduate level because although they may argue that they are using humour and sharing self with their patients, they need to consider care-fully whether this type of interaction is patient-focused or self-focused. Talking about their personal and social lives and using humour with patients is important in helping students to relax around patients and establish relationships with them. Patients also often enjoy these interactions, which may help to alleviate the boredom of hospital life. However, nursing students need to be mindful as they try to develop their confidence and communication skills, that the focus of interactions with patients should always be the patient. This does not mean that you should not talk about yourself, in fact, when you first meet a patient, it is often necessary to talk about yourself first in order to make the patient feel comfortable. So talking to a patient about where you come from, your family and even your social life may seem like a social conversation and, therefore, perhaps not that important. However, it provides the nurse with the opportunity to ask the patient about himself or herself and helps the nurse to establish a rapport with the patient and try to determine their needs. For the patient, this type of conversation gives them the opportunity to decide if the nurse is a good person and if they trust them or not. It also provides normal social interactions that patients often miss when they are in hospital.

Nurse-focused, first-level responses include, guarding, dehumanizing, withdrawing, distancing, labelling and denying often delivered using the 'busy nurse' persona. These can be a conscious or unconscious response that nurses use to detach from difficult or emotional situations in an effort to overcome stress or very intense feelings. The difficulty with this type of communication is that it can be over used because it allows nurses to get their work done with minimal emotional distraction. However, it can result in isolating patients and making them feel anxious and lonely.

Nurse-focused, second-level communication includes rote or mechanical response, false pity and false reassurance. Nurses who communicate in this way can appear distant and uncaring to their patients and this can make patients feel undervalued as individuals. This lowers their self-esteem and may prevent them from trusting the nurses and talking to the nurses about how they are feeling, either physically or psychologically. As nurses, phrases like 'Don't worry' and 'Everything will be fine' tend to come easily but they fall under the heading of the nurse-focused, second-level communication or false-reassurance even if they are spoken with the best of intentions.

Statements like these to patients can make them feel that they are over-reacting to their own illness or possibly that nobody is interested in their worries or fears. Nurses may use these responses unconsciously to prevent the patient from verbalizing any further fears. This is because the emotions that are evident in the patient or those that the nurse may start to feel are too difficult or intense to deal with or they may feel that they do not have time to listen and then deal with the issues that the patient raises.

This model of communication developed by Morse et al. (1992) (Figure 1.2) is quite a comprehensive model for nursing as it relates to many nursing contexts and disciplines. For example, it is applicable to areas such as day surgery or emergency nursing where the nurse-patient relationship is transient and its duration is limited. It is also relevant in areas where the nurse-patient relationship is long-term, for example long-stay units, residential homes or when caring for chronically or terminally ill patients. This model is particularly useful for helping nurses identify what communication responses constitute patient-focused communication and those that constitute nurse-focused communication. As previously mentioned, patient-focused, first-level emotion-based responses such as pity, sympathy and compassion are often undervalued in nursing whereas concepts that offer a detached, more controlling approach to communication such as therapeutic empathy and counselling are often referred to as essential communication skills for nurses. These skills are derived from counselling theory and require very specific skills to be used by counsellors in very controlled atmospheres that focus on facilitating clients to find solutions for their problems. These concepts will be developed further in Chapter 4 when we talk about helping skills and empathy.

Morse et al. (1997) devised 'The Comforting Interaction-Relationship Model' based on nurse-patient interaction as a strategy for the nurse and the patient to establish a therapeutic relationship through negotiation. This model proposed that the primary goal of nursing is to help patients reach an acceptable comfort level while receiving essential nursing care. This model reflects aspects of the circular transactional model and the skills model of communication and it is an important model for nurses as it is patient-centred and recognizes that nurse–patient interactions and relationships are dynamic and guided by the context in which they occur. This model utilizes Peplau's (1952: 9) definition of 'relationship' as 'two persons come to know each other well enough to face the problems at hand in a cooperative way'. This means that even very short duration nurse–patient interactions can be regarded as relationships even though the nurse and patient may have only just met. Morse et al. (1997) identified three components to the model: nursing actions, patient actions and the evolving relationship.

Nursing actions occur simultaneously are interactive and consist of:

- Comforting strategies such as touch and listening that can be planned or subconscious, direct or indirect actions but to be successful they must be patient-centred, that is, used in response to a patient cue. An example of this is if a patient winces because they are in pain, then the nurse speaks softly and uses gentle touch.
- Styles of care that relate the use of a combination of particular comfort strategies.
- Patterns of relating that are learned professional behaviours using a combination of styles of care. As nurses become socialized and gain more experience, they use standardized and normative patterns of relating. These patterns vary depending on the nursing speciality and the nurses' role, for example, nurses working in emergency departments will use a different way of relating and behaving to nurses working in community care.

Patient actions are:

- Signals of discomfort that can be verbal, non-verbal, situational or environmental, for example, a patient may state that they are experiencing pain or they may indicate by constantly shifting in the bed that they are in pain or they find it difficult to sleep because of noise around them during the day or night.
- Indices of distress emerge from signals of discomfort that a patient may give and they indicate that the patient needs a

nursing intervention, for example, pre-operatively a patient may appear agitated, restless, wringing their hands. By talking to the patient and reassuring them, the nurse can reduce the patient's level of stress.

- Patterns of relating to a nurse are only developed when a patient decides whether or not they trust the nurse and relinquish to care or reject nursing interventions. At this stage in the relationship, the patient controls the response of the nurse and the nature of the subsequent relationship. This means that this model recognizes that the patient has ultimate control in the type of relationship that develops between the nurse and patient.

The evolving relationship is the third component of this model and it describes nursing and patient actions as the means by which the nurse–patient relationship is negotiated by the nurse and patient and subsequently develops. Nurses respond to patient signals of discomfort and indices of distress using comforting strategies, styles of caring and patterns of relating on an ongoing and changing basis.

One important aspect to nurse–patient communication, and you may have noticed this already, is its 'unconscious' nature. Often our communication with others is unconscious, that is, we have many interactions with people but usually we do not plan them or think about the outcome. How then can nurses be certain that the way they communicate is patient-centred? Berry (2009) and Kruijver et al. (2001) suggest that nurses regularly use the linear model of one-way communication when caring for patients and the reasons for this have already been alluded to. They often profess to be too busy to deal with the unexpected and possibly difficult concerns that patients may have or they may feel that they just do not have the time to actually listen. One-way communication allows nurses to control the interaction and when nurses feel that they have a lot of work to do or tasks to complete, this is a useful way of communicating. However, the consequence of this type of communication is that it does not recognize the patient as the centre of care but rather the nurses need to complete the task takes precedence over the needs of the patient. Interestingly McCabe (2004), Chan et al. (2012) and Jakobsson and

Holmberg (2012) argued that patient-centred communication does not necessarily take up more of the nurses' time, it is not, they suggested, an additional task for the nurse. Rather it is simply portrayed by nurses in the words and body language that they choose to use when approaching patients. This notion, and its relationship to the concept of patient-centred communication forms the basis of Morse et al.'s (1997) model and will be discussed in greater detail in Chapter 3.

Exercise

Before you read the next chapter ask yourself the following questions:

- In what situations am I most aware of how I communicate at work?
- In what situations am I most aware of how I communicate in my personal life?
- Are these situations where I am striving to meet my own needs?

When you have written down your answers read them back and ascertain whether or not they reflect a patient-centred approach to care.

Key points

- We communicate because as human beings, we are compelled to.
- The way we, as individuals, communicate influences the type of relationship we have with others.
- Communication in nursing is concerned with providing individualized nursing care and coordinating interdisciplinary care in a patient-centred way.
- Communication is a complex, dynamic process that often occurs outside a person's awareness.
- In order for communication to be effective and patient-centred, nurses need to develop awareness of how they communicate and the influence this has on the nurse–patient relationship.
- Good communication is not more time consuming than bad communication.

2 Nursing Theory

Introduction

Now that we have given some explanation in the first chapter about communication theory, we are going to look a little bit more closely at the overall theoretical foundation of nursing care in order to examine and more fully understand where communication and communication theory fit into this. Within this context we will give consideration to person-centred holistic models of care in the healthcare setting and how these can influence communication and also facilitate inter-professional and inter-agency working.

Theoretical underpinnings of nursing

One prime motivator for the development of nursing theory in recent decades is the belief that although nurses work in parallel with many other healthcare professionals, they assess, plan, implement and evaluate care in their own right. Therefore, striving towards developing a unified body of knowledge that would inform and direct nursing care occurred within the context of the professionalization of nursing. This prompted nurse academics to explore nursing theory as a suitable evidence base for nursing practice.

In this chapter we examine theories of nursing and outline how they may be used in nursing practice to enhance nurse–patient communication. This knowledge of specific nursing theory will help to build on definitions of communication developed in the previous chapter. Although the nursing theories presented have unique foci upon nursing care, their emphasis on communication within the healthcare setting and nurse–patient relationship is common to all. There is a common belief among theorists that communication within a nurse–patient relationship is a fundamental aspect of nursing care delivery. We consider the relative importance of communication and discuss the importance of views of communication and the impact that this may have on patient outcome.

What is nursing theory?

> **Exercise**
>
> Describe your *theory* of nursing (what nursing is) in two to three lines.

You may well have described nursing as caring or in terms of nursing actions such as taking blood pressure and pulse measurements, or patient hygiene. If so your theory of nursing is quite similar to those developed by nurse theorists, although theirs, at first glance appear more complex.

> **Exercise**
>
> From your description of nursing *theory* above outline nurses' actions (what nurses do) in two to three lines.

Hopefully you will see from this exercise that how you perceive nursing (your theory) influences how you describe that role. For example, if you see nursing as caring, then the actions you describe will have a caring focus. If you see nursing as a series of physical tasks, then the actions will also reflect this. This is the basis for nursing theory development. By specifically encouraging nurses to see nursing in a particular way it is hoped to influence nursing actions in a positive way.

More specifically many theories of nursing aimed to move nursing away from a primarily task-focused occupation. Accounts of nursing practice up until the 1990s was often focused on completion of various tasks (Jenner 1998). Focusing on tasks (such as measuring urine output) allowed the nursing to be completed satisfactorily and was central to the role (Melia 1998). In addition this 'task orientation' as it is known (Jenner 1998: 1092) is thought to be a coping strategy used by nurses to avoid the emotional burden of caregiving (Martin 1998). In modern nursing this focus on tasks has been replaced with a greater focus on the individual patient's needs, and responding to each individual in a unique way. This approach is central to many of the developing theories.

Exercise

Consider for a moment the effects (on patients) of nursing practice that is task driven rather than individualized to patients. Write two to three lines.

From your response you will probably have identified that patients themselves may feel.

Exercise

Think for a moment how you would feel in the following situation.

How do you think the patients feel in the situation? Write two to three lines.

You are a student nurse working on a busy medical ward. You are new to this ward as it is only your second day. To speed up the morning's work your mentor asks you to carry out the blood pressure monitoring of the 12 patients in your care that day. You proceed to do this, greeting each patient in the ward by name and explaining the task that you need to carry out.

In the above scenario you might have felt that carrying out this task in this way left you little time to discuss the results fully with patients. Or perhaps you were conscious that patients may realize that you have jobs to be done and may not wish to disturb you with questions or queries. You may have identified that patients may feel that you are not directing your care to them as a person; rather you are concerned with getting the job done. Indeed this is exactly what happens in these circumstances. Patients even if their contact with the healthcare situation is short like to feel that they are known as individuals by staff and also treated in a person centred way (Costa 2001). This includes being referred to by name but also to the way in which nursing care is carried out, as one patient outlines:

> Probably, my biggest fear is like, when the nurse is there that she is really treating me, and treating me as a whole person, not just one more person to get in and get out. And not feeling like a cattle factory. That is very important to me. (Costa 2001: 879)

Similarly McCabe (2004) found that when patients saw nurses occupied with tasks like blood pressure they did not want to disturb them or take them from these jobs. However, while the busyness of the clinical situation would seem to prevent you as a student being responsive in an individualized way, studies show that the presence that patients require from the nurse doesn't have to be time consuming (McCabe 2004; Costa 2001). Quite straightforward communication skills make a big difference to patients' experience (Timmins et al. 2005). Calling patients by name, and a wave with a smile are just two examples of simple communication measures that can be used to ensure that communication is more patient centred (McCabe 2004; Timmins et al. 2005). Further examples include:

> she'd say 'how are you today John? ... it's things like that that help to cheer you up, particularly when you're in hospital' (McCabe 2004: 43).

> There was one particular girl, she was lovely ... every morning she'd come in and ask how you were or if she was going by she'd wave in to you (McCabe 2004: 46)

These gestures, however small they may seem, can demonstrate the genuine reflexive level of patient-focused communication that is discussed in Chapter 1. Conversely a focus on tasks may actually be inadvertently used by staff to guard or shield against direct patient contact. This is in keeping with the self-focused professional communication discussed in Chapter 1, that is a 'professional distancing' (Martin, 1998: 193) that takes place and no longer has the patient as the centre of care.

Exercise

Have you noticed occasions where individualized nursing care did not occur? Can you identify possible reasons for this?
    Write two to three lines.

Over time task repetition in nursing can ultimately become a ritual nursing action. This means that these tasks or patterns of behaviours are carried out repeatedly without thoughtful purpose or reconsidering their necessity or their evidence base. Assessing patients' body temperature, for example, is one area where risk of ritual was predicted as far back as the 1970s:

> temperature recording ... is so much a part of the everyday routine of practising nurses that it stands in danger of becoming more of a ritual than a useful observation of a patient (Sims-Williams 1976: 481)

In the past it was found that nurses took recordings of temperature in a ritualistic fashion (every six hours) when often the patients' condition did not warrant this. Indeed as recently as 2011, ritualistic actions related to both nurses' assessment and treatment are observed (Thompson and Kagan 2011). This notion of ritualistic or task-oriented care, although perceived as predominately a feature of the past, is also potential feature of new nursing roles. Expanding nurse roles within Europe such as specialist nurse and advanced nurse practitioner (Riley et al. 2003), as they are often not standardized and are unregulated, run the risk of becoming comprising the performance of junior doctor's tasks instead of advancing the role of nursing in healthcare (Thompson 2002). Thompson (2002: 8) also highlights that 'there is a danger that [in these roles] nurses focus solely on particular aspects of medical treatment rather than focus on the totality of patient care'.

This use of rituals affects the nurse's ability to communicate effectively (Martin 1998). Rather than an open communication system Martin (1998) suggested that communication rituals are socially constructed within the healthcare setting, and communication during nursing procedures is often a condensed and restricted, and ultimately a, source of patient control, rather than a therapeutic intervention. Furthermore, this ritualistic communication is 'full of jargon and abbreviations impossible for those outside the profession to understand' (Martin, 1998: 189).

The nature of ritualistic communication is unlikely to be patient centred as it serves the purpose of the nurse. Rituals, Martin (1998) proposes, has its basis in a task-orientated approach to nursing care. Despite rhetoric of patient centred care, the focus of many hospital wards is getting the work done. Martin (1998:193) suggests that this 'contributes to the "busy nurse" syndrome which keeps the nurse active all the time and protects him/her from the need to talk to the patient'. This busyness allows the nurse to legitimately distance themselves from patients thus allowing no time for nurse-patient interaction'. This has obvious potential repercussions for nurse patient communication.

Exercise

List and identify nursing rituals that you may have encountered. Identify possible reasons for these.

Patient centred communication is not only good for patients it is also good for the healthcare system. In the United States one comparison of doctor's malpractice claim histories revealed that patient-centred communication practices were associated with less claims (Wissow 2004).

Patient centredness requires recognition of the uniqueness of the individual; it requires core communication skills and individual patient needs assessment. These items are central components of nursing theory and conceptual model use in nursing. Therefore, we will examine theories of nursing and outline how they may be used in nursing practice to enhance nurse–patient communication and the therapeutic relationship, by fostering holistic nursing care. This knowledge of specific nursing theory will help to build on definitions of communication developed in the previous chapter.

Using nursing theory in practice

Using nursing theory to guide this nursing practice requires the use of a suitable theoretical framework with which to conceptualize, describe and inform the unique contribution of the nurse in healthcare settings. The terms conceptual models and theory are often used interchangeably, and while many theorists outline both a theory and a conceptual model, significant differences exist in the definition and understanding of both (Fawcett 2005). Practicing nurses are most familiar with the use of conceptual models. These are but one component of that which Fawcett (2005) referred to as a structural hierarchy of knowledge in nursing:

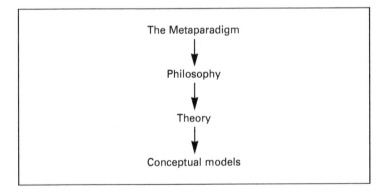

In Fawcett's hierarchy the most abstract level of knowledge is the metaparadigm. This identifies overarching concepts under consideration. In nursing, these are the person, the environment, health and nursing (Alligood 2006a). The metaparadigm does not provide direct guidance to practice, but rather presents a broad view of the uniform understandings within a discipline that inform the theory.

Philosophy, the second component in the hierarchy, is a statement of beliefs (Kim 1983). Each theory of nursing has its own philosophy that informs the theory. The theory itself, although abstract, guides and informs nursing practice. Conceptual models of nursing represent the final aspect of the knowledge hierarchy. They provide frameworks to guide and direct nursing care. Each conceptual model provides a unique direction to nursing practice (Fawcett 2005).

The potential contribution of nursing theory to guide communication practice in nursing

The emergence and continued development of nursing theory and conceptual models to guide practice, which occurred mostly in the United States, has become synonymous with the individualization of patient care. It also serves to reduce the use of ritual, routine, task orientation and use of the medical model through the promotion of thoughtful, insightful care planning for each individual patient (Alligood 2006b). Nursing theory offers nursing a distinct scientific knowledge base to guide practice. Without the use of nursing theory to guide practice, rituals are likely to prevail. Although there have been, and continue to be, issues with nursing theory and conceptual model use, such as difficulty with relevance and application to practice and concerns about empirical testing and associated documentation, their overall contribution to the individualization of nursing is something that cannot be ignored in a consideration of factors that could improve the nurse–patient therapeutic relationship. In addition, as most nursing theory focuses on communication as a distinct aspect of the role of the nurse, it is important to explore the potential contribution of nursing theory and conceptual models of nursing to communication practice.

Nursing theory as a guide to communication behaviour in nursing

Nursing theory and conceptual model use to guide nurse–patient communication practices

Partnership in the nurse–patient relationship with recognition of patient autonomy is a recurring theme throughout popular nursing theory (Pearson et al. 2005). This particular aspect of nursing has particular relevance when moving away from the medical, traditional and routine models of care (Pearson et al. 2005). We selected theories for consideration in this chapter due to their popularity and relevance to the topic under consideration. These are the Roper-Logan-Tierney (RLT) conceptual model (Roper et al. 1980, 1985, 1990, 1996, 2001), Orem's Self-Care Deficit Theory of Nursing (SCDNT) (Orem 1971, 1980, 1985, 1991, 1995, 2001) and Peplau's Conceptual Frame of Reference for Psychodynamic Nursing (Peplau, 1952, 1991).

The Roper-Logan-Tierney model of nursing (RLT) (Roper et al. 1980, 1985, 1990, 1996, 2001) is a conceptual model and a theory of nursing that developed in Edinburgh. It is widely used throughout the United Kingdom and Ireland and internationally (Holland et al. 2008a:2) 'as a framework for nursing care and practice and teaching and learning'. The RLT accepts the uniqueness of each individual (Holland 2008). The individualization of care using RLT allows for the particular understanding of different cultures and language barriers that can exist when caring for patients (Holland et al. 2008b). This is especially so in today's multicultural environment.

Orem's Self-Care Deficit Nursing Theory (SCDNT) (Orem, 2001), is one of the most widely used theories in practice. Although primarily a theory of nursing, Fawcett (2005) noted that the concepts and propositions of this theory can also be used at a practical (conceptual model) level; and may be used therefore used as a framework to guide specific nursing actions. Peplau's Conceptual Frame of Reference for Psychodynamic Nursing (Peplau, 1952, 1991) is a theory of nursing.

It is beyond the scope of the chapter to describe these models in their totality and reference to seminal texts is advised. The Roper-Logan-Tierney model of nursing (RLT) was described in original texts (Roper et al. 1980, 1985, 1990, 1996, 2001) and other useful texts on the topic (Pearson et al. 2005, Holland et al. 2008). It is underpinned by a 'model of living' described by Roper et al. (2001) who identified five main components of human living that constituted the 'main features of this highly complex phenomenon'(13). These concepts are interrelated and comprise:

- Activities of living (ALs)
- Lifespan
- Dependence/independence continuum
- Factors influencing the ALs
- Individuality in living (Roper et al. 2001).

Roper et al. (2001) proposed that living involved the completion of 12 activities of living (ALs):

1. maintaining a safe environment;
2. communicating;
3. breathing;
4. eating and drinking;
5. eliminating;
6. personal cleansing and dressing;
7. controlling body temperature;
8. working and playing;
9. mobilizing;
10. sleeping;
11. expressing sexuality; and
12. dying.

These ALs are the central focus of the model. It was the interaction and relationship between the ALs and the other components (Figure 2.1) that facilitated the notion of individuality as a discrete component to emerge (Roper et al. 2001).

The nursing process (assess, plan, implement and evaluate) is used in conjunction with the RLT (Roper et al. 2001). Persons requiring nursing care undergo an assessment in each of the ALs with consideration of the factors influencing these activities, the dependence independence continuum and lifespan issues.

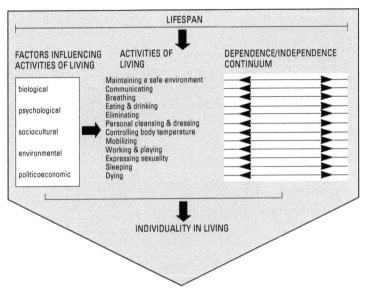

Figure 2.1   The model of living

Source: Roper, N., Logan, W. W. and Tierney, A. J. (2001) *The Roper Logan Tierney Model of Nursing Based on Activities of Living,* London: Churchill Livingstone. Reproduced with kind permission from Elsevier Ltd

Problems (actual or potential) are identified and transferred to a care plan, so that necessary nursing care may be planned, implemented and documented. At later stages of the nursing process the care given is evaluated. This process, which they describe as dynamic and continuous, is displayed in Figure 2.2.

Roper et al. (2001) emphasized the individual nature of this process of nursing and the necessity for patient participation, all elements of what we may begin to consider as patient-centred care. Their model also allows for specific assessment of individual needs and problems in the activity of communication (AL) and thus may be said to facilitate patient-centred communication. In their commentary on communication as an AL, Roper et al. (2001: 22) highlighted that this is 'a highly individual activity' however, 'it is not the individual who is crucial, but the interpersonal relationship' – introducing another important element in communication, the nurse–patient relationship.

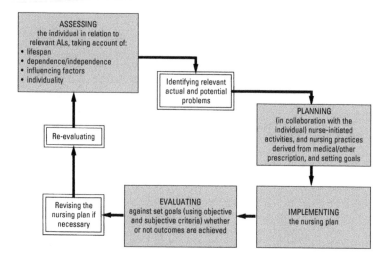

Figure 2.2 Individualizing nursing as a dynamic process using the Roper–Logan–Tierney Model of Nursing

Source: Roper, N., Logan, W. W. and Tierney, A. J. (2001) *The Roper Logan Tierney Model of Nursing Based on Activities of Living,* London: Churchill Livingstone. Reproduced with kind permission from Elsevier Ltd

Although description of the nature of the assessment for this activity emphasizes the individual nature of communication, there is little direction on the development of the nurse–patient relationship. The assessment focuses on identifying the usual pattern of communication factors (biological, psychological, sociocultural, environmental and politicoeconomic) affecting this activity (Pearson et al. 2005) and the identification of problems (Iggulden 2008).

The underlying assumptions of Orem's Self-Care Deficit Nursing Theory (SCDNT) (Orem 2001) include: that individuals require continuous personal and environmental input in order to function effectively; that human *agency* (the ability to act deliberately) involves self-care and care of others that is based upon needs; mature humans can experience limitations on this (self-care and care of others); this agency develops over time; and this agency enables oneself or others to provide inputs to ensure effective functioning.

The SCDNT incorporates three intertwining theories

(Orem 2001): self-care, self-care deficit and the theory of nursing systems. Self-care, Orem (2001) suggested, must be learned and performed deliberately. This theory assumes everyone develops and uses skills throughout their life to enable them to be able to take care of themselves and their dependents. The *theory of self-care deficit* explains that when people's needs for care exceed their own ability to meet these needs they may require nursing care.

The *theory of nursing systems* brings together all the essential components of the SCDNT. It explains that nursing is a human action formed by nurses through the exercise of their nursing agency for persons with health-derived or health-associated limitations in self-care or dependent care.

Therapeutic self-care is an essential element in the SCDNT. The nurse may assess therapeutic self-care demand by analyzing therapeutic self-care requisites in three distinct domains: universal, health deviation and developmental.

Universal self-care requisites are universally required goals that are met through self-care or dependent care. Eight self-care requisites common to all were identified by Orem (2001):

1. The maintenance of a sufficient intake of air.
2. The maintenance of a sufficient intake of water.
3. The maintenance of a sufficient intake of food.
4. The provision of care associated with elimination processes and excrements.
5. The maintenance of balance between activity and rest.
6. The maintenance of balance between solitude and social interaction.
7. The prevention of hazards to human life, human functioning, and human well-being.
8. The promotion of human functioning and development within social groups in accordance with human potential, known human limitations and the human desire to be normal.

Meeting the universal self-care requisites through self-care or dependent-care is an integral component of the daily living of individuals and groups.

A later addition to the model, *developmental self-care requisites* are concerned with all aspects of human development. Orem (2001) outlined three sets of developmental requisites: the provision of conditions that promote development, engagement in self-development, and interferences with development.

Health deviation self-care requisites are self-care requisites that exist for persons who are ill or injured, who have specific forms of pathological conditions or disorders and who are undergoing medical diagnosis treatment.

The first stage for nurses when using this model is *assessment*. This 'calculation and design' of the therapeutic self-care demand requires an 'investigative process' Orem (2001: 247). Although not explicitly stated in the model, the nursing process underpins the operation of the model in practice. This information is transferred to a care plan. *Planning* outlines the amount of care that an individual requires. It involves outlining the actions (related to human functioning and development) that the individual should perform or have performed by another within a specific timeframe.

Intervention involves nursing systems – a series of deliberate (collaborative with patient) practical actions to meet patients' therapeutic self-care demands and to protect and promote patients' self-care agency (ability to meet their own needs) (Orem 2001).

Within this nursing system, nursing care can be described and implemented on a continuum ranging from *wholly compensatory* (doing for the patient), *partly compensatory* (helping the patient to do for himself or herself) or *supportive-educative* (helping the patient learn to do for himself or herself).

Partnership is an explicit aspect of the use of SCNT as a conceptual model in practice. Empowerment is also crucial. Rather than nursing care being regarded solely as providing direct care to another Orem (2001) also highlighted the important nursing actions of supporting and educating patients. The development of the nurse–patient relationship was identified as crucial to this process (Orem 2001) as it is essential for the full and participative involvement of patients in care as suggested.

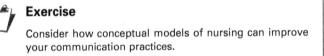

	Orientation	Identification	Exploitation	Resolution
Admission	••			
Intervention	••	••	••	
Recovery	••	••	••	••
Discharge			••	••

Figure 2.3 Overlapping phases in nurse–patient relationships

Source: Peplau (1991) *Interpersonal relations in Nursing a Conceptual Framework of Reference for Psychodynamc Nursing,* New York: Springer. Reproduced with permission of SPRINGER PUBLISHING COMPANY INC in the format republished in a book via Copyright Clearance Center.

Exercise

Consider how conceptual models of nursing can improve your communication practices.

The development of a nurse–patient relationship was a fundamental component of Peplau's (1952, 1991) work. This Conceptual Frame of Reference for Psychodynamic Nursing held that the emphasis in nursing care was the growth of the patient through partnership with the nurse. This partnership (nurse–patient relationship) evolves through distinct phases (Figure 2.3). During the orientation phase patients' individual communication needs are considered and addressed. Peplau (1991) specified nursing actions during this phase to include acting as a resource person, as a listener and as a technical expert. The patient begins to identify their needs from the experience.

Exercise

Consider how you may identify patients' needs during the orientation phase?

In the next phase, identification, the patient may strongly identify with a nurse as the basis for the formation of the nurse–patient relationship. Peplau (1991: 37) outlined how both the patient and nurse 'make use' of this identification. Both the nurse and patient allow this developing professional relationship to form the basis of recovery. Once this identification takes place, Peplau (1991) suggested that patients proceed to a phase (exploitation) whereby the patient 'makes full use of the services offered to him'. The patient should feel confident and able to utilize the resources available in the healthcare context. When goals have been achieved, resolution occurs and new goals are formed for discharge. Peplau (1991: 40) suggested that this phase will only occur through 'psychological mothering' and she described one role of the nurse as a 'surrogate'. While this language and thinking appears outdated, the fundamental message is not: that a 'sustaining relationship' (1991: 40) between nurses and patient that allows identification of individual patient needs and enables action to address these needs and provides emotional support is required. Other roles identified by Peplau (1991) were: counsellor, resource, teacher, technical expert and leader.

Exercise

Consider how you may increase the likelihood of patient identification with the nurse during this phase?

The importance of the nurse–patient relationship within nursing was of crucial importance to Peplau (1991). Pearson et al. (2005: 181) noted that in concentrating 'on developing the ideas of nursing and interpersonal processes she [Peplau] gives only cursory consideration to health and the environment'. The interpersonal relationship advocated by Peplau (1991) fosters patient recovery and rehabilitation but also allows 'individuals to understand their health problems and to learn from their experience' (Pearson et al. 2005: 181).

These notions are of particular relevance in today's healthcare setting. In a consumer-driven era there is increasing emphasis on patient satisfaction with services. Although in many cases the procedural aspects of hospitalized care may have been intact, the literature abounds with research indicating that communication within the healthcare setting is less than optimal. In addition, with the increasing use and publication of qualitative studies, there are many examples of the emotional consequences of hospitalization. Furthermore, there is increasing evidence that patients' educational needs are not always met in the hospital setting.

This model emphasizes and extends the development of the nurse–patient relationship, which should become, as it was for Peplau (1991) the main focus of care. For Peplau, the nurse–patient relationship and interaction (the interpersonal relationship) is the essence of nursing (Pearson et al. 2005). This one-to-one approach this may help to improve communication, information giving and emotional support given by nurses. Although there is a concern that over involvement at a personal level may occur, there is an emphasis on professional closeness (Pearson et al. 2005).

Peplau's (1991) theory of nursing is carried out through observation, communication and recording. The process is recorded in Figure 2.4. The development of the interpersonal relationship between patient and nurse, aimed at developing the patient, through the various phases identified, is a predominant theme in this book. It is helpful to understand the nurse–patient relationship as occurring in these four phases (orientation, identification, exploration and resolution) even within short interactions. Remember, although we are social beings interaction with patients, while it may have social elements such as greetings, is primarily a health goal driven professional, healing relationship (Arnold and Underman Boggs 2011). The ultimate goal is patient growth (see Figure 2.4). From a communication perspective the patient ought not to be harmed in any way by the interaction, but rather strengthened by it. This can be achieved through the personal approaches mentioned earlier in the chapter such as remembering and using the patient's name at all times during these four phases. During orientation and identification keeping the family involved is also important in many settings (Wheeler 2010), and building up a rapport with patients can be done in simple ways for example, while helping

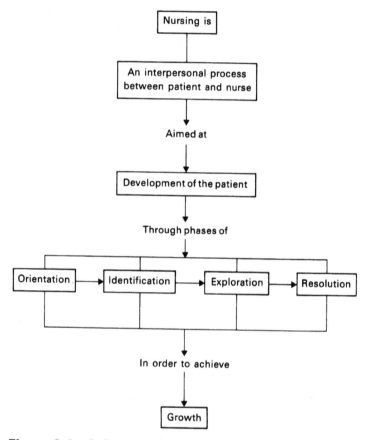

Figure 2.4 A diagramatic representation of Peplau's developmental model

Source: Pearson, A, Vaughan.B. and Fitzgerald M. (2005) *Nursing Models for Practice*, 3rd edn, London: Butterworth Heinemann. Reproduced with kind permission from Elservier Ltd (Butterworth Heinemann)

with dressing by 'picking up a picture and saying, '"Oh, who's this?" And talking about that person' (Wheeler 2010: 19). The notion of therapeutic communication is continued and developed in the next chapter.

As a student you may become familiar with using a conceptual model of nursing during your clinical placements. Organizations usually choose one conceptual model of nursing, suited to their philosophy in order to guide and direct nursing care. This is also used to underpin nursing documentation. One site can choose to use a single model or to use a combination of approaches.

Exercise

Identify the conceptual model of nursing used in an area where you work or study.

You may find from your examination of the documentation used at the site that the conceptual model varies a little from that presented above. This is because clinical staff are encouraged to adapt these models to suit the local environment. The Nottingham model (Smith 1995) for example, that is used widely in children's nursing is an adaptation of the RLT model discussed above although it is also thought to have been influenced by Orem's SCDNT (Lee 2003). Approaches to nursing based on the RLT are also common in the United Kingdom, and if you are working in the United Kingdom you are likely to come across this.

Exercise

If you come across approaches to nursing care based on the RLT model identify the approaches to communication used. Write two to three lines.
Identify whether or not the patients' level of communication is assessed and how.
Identify whether or not the RLT model guides your communication.

While you may find variations in approach, it is likely that the RLT specifically guides communication mostly through the use of documentation. At a basic level this documentation gives you both a language and an approach to use in your nursing care. You will see that you are provided you with specific words to use (such as the ALs outlined above) within the context of a specific approach to nursing care (the nursing process), which differs according to and takes account of changes in lifespan (Iggulden 2008). Thus, you will notice first that communication is considered seriously within the framework of a holistic patient assessment and second that as a nurse RLT provides you with some vocabulary to guide your own communication, in addition to guiding overall approaches to care.

Although perhaps not explicit from the documentation that you have viewed, or your experiences in nursing, the RLT expressly guides nurses' assessment of patients' communication needs and abilities. First biological, psychological, sociocultural and environmental issues may need to be taken into account during this assessment (Iggulden 2008). Other diagnostic tools such as the Glasgow Coma Scale may also be used in this assessment, if the patient has sustained a head injury or has other neurological damage (Iggulden 2008). Assessing the patient's level of understanding and writing ability is also useful to the assessment (Iggulden 2008). Consider the following case study:

Darvesh Daswani is a 58 year old man admitted with a right sided hemiparesis (weakness) and dysphasia (difficulty speaking). His condition is currently stable undergoing tests to establish his underlying diagnosis. He is married with three adult children who live nearby.

Exercise

What approaches you would take when assessing Darvesh's AL specifically related to the activity of communication?
What kinds of questions could you ask to help make a nursing assessment of [Darvesh's] communication needs and abilities?' (Iggulden 2008: 106).
Using RLT as a basis to plan care, identify three main items that would form the basis of the care plan (ADL of communication)?
What approaches would you use to communicate with Darvesh?

Hopefully you will see from this case study example above that conceptual models of care, derived from nursing theory are helpful in guiding approaches to communication with patients in your care. You will find similar approaches adopted by other models of care that are in use in practice. In some clinical areas there is a move away from traditional care plan use as nurses often did not find these very useful. They found that they involved a lot of paperwork with little evidence of benefits to the patients (Griffiths 1998; Mason 1999; Murphy et al. 2000). Furthermore one recent analysis outlined problems with conceptual models' relevance to nursing, their lack of specific direction for care and their lack of congruency with working with an evidence base (McCrae 2012). Thus, you may come across a range of alternative approaches to care in practice such as multidisciplinary care pathways or person-centred plans. However, regardless of the approaches to care used a mental model of care is often in use by nurses (Wimpenny 2001) either influenced directly by the approach to care advocated in the healthcare setting, or based on their own experience. It is hoped from your reading of this chapter and your growing understanding of communication skills that your mental image will have a strong focus on the importance of both assessing and responding to patients communication needs and your own use of good communication skills.

Despite the criticism of nursing theory and conceptual model use in nursing, their use over a number of years has contributed to attempts to move away from task-orientated nursing to individualized patient-centred care. As patient-focused nursing actions are key to good communication in nursing, the use of conceptual models of nursing or approaches to care that foster individualized care, are a good support in developing and maintaining good nurse–patient communication mechanisms. Nurses need to 'communicate safely and effectively with patients and their families' (An Bord Altranais 2010: 6) and nursing theory/conceptual model use, through individualized care plans, is a vehicle for this. Furthermore as communication with patients ought to be health goal oriented and purposeful (rather than social) (Arnold and Underman Boggs 2011) using the nursing process for the basis of the relationship is useful. Ultimately what is required is a 'respectful culture' (Paton 2009:145). The Nursing and Midwifery Council state that: 'All nurses must use excellent communication and interpersonal skills. Their communications must always be safe, effective compassionate and respectful' (2010: 15)

Frameworks for nursing care delivery that encompass a specific focus on communication such as those discussed above are a useful conduit to ensure that professional therapeutic patient-centred relationships develop in the context of holistic, multidisciplinary patient care. Furthermore Peplau's (1952, 1991) conceptual model of the nurse–patient relationship is a useful adjunct to nursing model use. You can use this personally to develop and reflect upon your own communication skills, but also as a frame of reference for your communications in practice. The Tidal Model (Barker 2001) used within the mental health settings (Ward and Jackson 2006) is an adaptation and development of Peplau's work (Barker 2001). This is a good working example of how this theory can be put into use in practice, and used to support and develop therapeutic nurse–patient relationships. While this specific use of a conceptual model use is more concerned with multidisciplinary and patient involvement in specific settings (mental health) it is important to note that patient centredness and good communication skills remain central principles of model use, thus emphasizing the importance of these concepts.

Conclusion

Communication is recognized and accepted as both a fundamental process within the domain of healthcare required for effective management of care and service delivery (Notara et al. 2010). Patient safety and quality are key components of contemporary healthcare delivery and effective communication is a crucial component of these (HIQA 2010). Through a brief exploration of nursing theory and conceptual models and their potential contribution to care it is obvious that this conceptualization of nursing represents a step forward in the holistic care of patients by nurses. As, by their nature they consider the individual, health, nursing and the environment, they have made an immeasurable contribution towards the individualization of nursing. Furthermore, their focus on communication skills and the nurse–patient relationship as a core component of nursing has important implications.

Roper et al. (2001) suggested a very individualized approach to nursing with special consideration for communication ability/problems of the patient. Orem (2001) emphasized patient empowerment and self-care and the important role that the nurse–patient relationship has in fostering this. Peplau (1991) focused almost exclusively on the nurse–patient relationship with an unparalleled suggestion of the therapeutic contribution of this relationship. Description of these models in this chapter illuminates the importance that nurse theorists place on not only communication skills of nurses, but also assessment skills and relationship building. The use of each of these approaches to care will influence care management in different ways. However, fundamental to these approaches is the developing notion of therapeutic communication and patient-centred communication. It is only through the adoption of these principles that current gaps in service provision can be addressed and healthcare provision can become truly customer orientated and based on community and individual needs.

Key points

▶ Nursing theory can be used as a framework to conceptualize, describe and inform the unique contribution of nursing to healthcare provision.

▶ Nursing theory and conceptual model use guides and informs nursing practice, thus, preventing ritualistic nursing.

▶ The integral role of communication and patient-centredness is a recurring theme in contemporary nursing theory that provides a nursing rather than task–oriented model of care.

▶ Nurses need to consider personal approaches to patient-centred communication within the context of particular approaches to nursing care delivery.

3 Effective Communication

Introduction

This chapter explores the concepts of therapeutic and patient-centred communication as effective mechanisms for communication in nursing practice. Psychological theories are introduced as a framework to develop the discussion and consideration of effective communication. These theories are commonly used by nurses to provide explanations about human behaviour. Having a greater awareness of what motivates a human to react in the way they do provides nurses with a greater understanding of patients in their care and when applied to the nurse–patient relationship. Within the context of healthcare, it is important to remember that the nurse is responsible for the relationship that develops. It is not a social relationship, determined by how well you might like or get along with a person, but a professional therapeutic relationship that needs to be effective in both supporting patients and their families and providing them with information. In some cases psychological theory allows you to see why a patient behaves in the way they do. Knowledge of these theories can also help nurses, as individuals and professionals, to understand their own behaviour in the nurse–patient relationship by helping them become aware of themselves, their personal needs and personal reactions.

Communication influences

Communication is a complex process involving both interpersonal and intrapersonal factors. Each person is a unique individual with a unique interpretation of the world influenced by origin, upbringing and life experience. (Hindle 2006: 53)

This statement outlines how factors within the person (intrapersonal) and between individuals (interpersonal) affect how we communicate. If we consider some of the 'noise' (DeVito 2011) that interferes with communication, some of this noise arises from intrapersonal factors: what is going on inside a person's head. Arnold and Underman Boggs (2011) termed this the 'internal frame of reference'. This is the personal lens through which each of us views the world. Communication influencing factors are:

- physical,
- environmental,
- socio-cultural, and
- psychological.

Both nurse and patient are influenced by:

- communication abilities,
- internal frame of reference,
- culture and role,
- knowledge, and
- psychological factors.

Psychological factors

Indeed DeVito (2011) specifically indentified 'psychological noise' as: 'a mental interference in speaker or listener and includes preconceived ideas, wandering thoughts, biases and prejudices, closed-mindedness, and extreme emotionalism'.

A range of psychological factors are thought to affect human behaviours. Hindle (2006) outlined a range of these:

- stage of maturation (development),
- defence mechanisms,
- attitudes and beliefs,
- assumptions and prejudices,
- perceptual distortions,
- mental illness and
- irrational beliefs (Arnold and Underman Boggs 2011).

These are best understood by exploring a range of classical psychological theories.

Sigmund Freud

The first of these theories relates to the work of Sigmund Freud who developed a model of personality that identified the *id*, the *ego* and the *superego* as the three main components of personality. The *id*, which is believed to be present at birth, is based on the pleasure principle. It represents the basic human need to satisfy certain desires, such as food, comfort and sleep in order to survive. The *ego* develops as the infant grows in response to its environment and is based on the reality principle. In other words it balances the drive of the *id* in the context of reality, what is socially acceptable behaviour and in maintaining self-esteem. The *superego* is the third and perhaps most complex aspect to the development of personality that begins to develop as the child becomes an adolescent. It is concerned with the development of conscience and the incorporation of an individual's and society's sense of morality and forms the basis of values and beliefs that play an integral role in behaviour. Freud believed essentially that unconscious forces and desires drive human behaviour and these need to become conscious so that healthy relationships can occur (Arnold and Underman Boggs 2011). While this detail may seem unrelated to explaining nurse–patient relationships, it does provide knowledge about human behaviour, the development of self through interaction with others and personal development (Arnold and Underman Boggs 2011). This in turn encourages and facilitates nurses to develop an awareness of the various forces that influence nurse–patient relationships and in particular how their personal behaviour contributes to the relationship and whether or not it is a therapeutic relationship for the patient.

Freud believed that human behaviour and decision making is unconsciously influenced by each individual's past experiences, feelings, values and beliefs. Freud introduced the concepts of transference and counter-transference as a means of explaining the underlying dynamic in an interaction

(Arnold and Underman Boggs 2011). Transference, which is also sometimes referred to as projection, is described as behaviour in which individuals unconsciously project seemingly inappropriate or irrational feelings/attitudes towards others that are based on previous personal experiences or relationships. In the context of the nurse–patient relationship this means, for example, that a patient communicates with a nurse based on a past relationship or experience that is unrelated to the present situation. Talking to a nurse may arouse feelings of anger in a patient whose has unresolved issues in relation to the death of a parent.

Counter-transference is the nurse's counter-reaction to the patient's transference and perhaps includes the nurses own transference issues. Transference and counter-transference is clearly a two-way process in which a person transfers or projects their own thoughts, feelings, emotions and needs onto another person either consciously or unconsciously. This can result in a positive or negative interaction but ultimately, and depending on the nature of the transference or counter-transference behaviours, it can influence the development of a therapeutic nurse–patient relationship.

Recognition of personal responses as counter-transference represents a challenge for nurses as does the understanding of the possible impact of these responses on the development of the nurse–patient relationship. Once a patient is labelled as 'difficult' it means that from the nurse's perspective, they become the reason why the nurse–patient relationship is a negative one. This of course is not the case but it is only by examining their own behaviour and developing an awareness of transference and counter-transference responses that they use, that nurses can begin to have a clearer picture of how they can ensure that the relationships that they have with patients, regardless of their duration, can be therapeutic.

Exercise

Think about one aspect of your parents' personality that evokes either positive or negative feelings in you. How does this part of their personality make you feel? Write a couple of lines.

> Next, think about a friend or partner and whether or not there is a link between a particular aspect of their personality that you react most strongly to and the one you identified in your parents. Write 2 to 3 lines
>
> You may see a link immediately but if not, think about whether or not you have the same response and reaction to other people who exhibit the same aspect of personality as your parents. This is transference.

This type of exercise may help you to develop awareness about your personal behaviour and realize that often the way we respond to others is often more about ourselves than those we are communicating with.

Maslow

In contrast to Freud, psychologists from the humanistic school of thought, such as, Maslow (1954) and Rogers (1961) were of the view that people are driven by positive forces to achieve their full potential in life. People are thought to be basically good and trustworthy and prefer growth and love to aggression and destruction. In order to understand human behaviour, individuals need to be considered as a whole rather than trying to understand humans as a combination of parts. Maslow (1954) believed that humans have specific needs that drive them towards ultimately meeting and satisfying these needs. These needs are described as a hierarchy with physiological needs (food, water, sleep being the most basic) that are present at birth. As the infant grows to childhood and then to adulthood their needs develop to include: safety, the need to belong, the need for a positive self-esteem and finally the need for self-actualization. In order to reach this a person would need to have achieved fulfilment in the other stages.

According to Maslow (1954) very few people achieve self-actualization, which he describes as a 'journey' or way of life rather than a goal in life. In his research Maslow was concerned with identifying things that make humans different from each other. In terms of nursing practice, this theory is useful for explaining or determining when a patient is ready for a nursing intervention. For example, if a nurse needs to change a dressing on a wound, they will ensure that the patient feels comfortable, warm, secure and pain free prior to starting the dressing. Throughout the procedure the nurse talks to the patient about the progress of wound healing and answers any queries the patient may have. Following the procedure the nurse will discuss when the next dressing needs to be done and what activities the patient can do in the meantime to promote wound healing. The nurse will leave the patient feeling comfortable and secure.

Carl Rogers

Roger's (1961) personality theory focuses on self-perception and self-concept as key aspects to understanding a person's personality and these emerge from interacting with others and feedback from others. He proposed that, unlike Freud's theory, human behaviour is purposeful: individuals are free to make choices and develop their own personalities rather than being driven by unconscious forces or learned behaviour. Rogers (1961) also adapts the humanistic approach and introduces the 'person-centred' theory.

This theory is concerned with understanding interpersonal interaction and Rogers (1961) identifies three key components of the person-centred theory. These are warmth, empathy and genuineness. Warmth is necessary for a relationship to develop and it refers to making an individual 'special' or that you respect them as an individual. To do this successfully, a person would need to exhibit unconditional positive regard towards others. This means having an innate respect for people that is non-judgmental. Empathy, which is regarded as a helping skill, will be discussed in detail in Chapter 4. Genuineness is a concept that is difficult to describe. It is a perception that a person has about another because they perceive that person to communicate in an open, honest and sensitive manner.

These qualities are imparted through the use of congruent behaviour, that is, the verbal language that a person uses matches their non-verbal language. This is the foundation stone of a therapeutic nurse–patient relationship. Some nurses find it easy to use these skills others may not. It can be a challenge to disregard our own views and feelings when caring for patients and accept them as unique individuals regardless of their background or illness. When a nurse labels a patient or passes judgment on them they will be unable to communicate in a therapeutic or patient-centred way because they are focusing on their own views and feelings rather than the needs of the patient as a unique individual.

Martin Buber

Martin Buber (1958) presented the view that our reality is defined by the way we speak to each other. He suggests that people use two ways of communicating: I-It and I-Thou. The I-It relationship occurs when we view people and issues objectively. An example of this in nursing is when a patient is described as 'the fractured hip in bed four'. Instead of sharing ourselves with patients, understanding them and talking to them as individuals, nurses consider it important to keep a 'distance' between themselves and the patients that they care for.

It is a relationship that demonstrates separateness and detachment. In contrast, the I-thou relationship is one of mutuality and reciprocity. In the nurse–patient relationship this means that the nurse and the patient respect each other as individuals with equal commitment and responsibility in the relationship. The individualized approach to nursing care as advocated by nurse theorists is in keeping with this theory, however, according to Buber (1958) each person needs to enter the I-Thou relationship without preconditions.

This can be a challenge for nurses because of how they are socialized. Traditionally nurses were not supported or encouraged by healthcare organizations to establish therapeutic relationships with patients. One possible reason for this is to reduce staff stress levels by encouraging nurses to distance themselves from difficult emotional situations. It seems that although nurses are no longer encouraged to distance themselves from patients, this practice remains in nursing culture.

Also just as nurses are socialized, patients too are socialized and have preconceived stereotyped ideas of the role of the nurse.

Patients, depending on their past experiences of being a patient, level of education, knowledge or personal views on health and illness, may wish to be active participants in planning and organizing their care. On the other hand some patients may take on a passive role and rely on the nurses and other healthcare professionals to make decisions regarding their care. However, an awareness by nurses of their own and possibly patients' preconceived ideas may compensate for this and by entering into the relationship with the I-Thou attitude or even Rogers patient-centred view then nurses may be able to use their communication skills to establish what level of control a patient wishes to have over every aspect of their care. For example, a patient may retain the role of meeting their own hygiene needs and actively discuss their illness and plan of care with the nurse but may resist giving their own insulin injection.

It requires sensitivity and empathy on the part of the nurse to recognize when a patient is not comfortable participating in their own care and provide an opportunity for the patient to verbalize their concerns and fears about participating. By providing opportunities where patients feel comfortable about voicing their concerns and do not feel a nuisance or that they are holding up the busy nurse, nurses will be able to provide more effective nursing care where the advice and education that they give to patients is individualized and meets the specific needs of the patient.

Psychological factors: anxiety

Another psychological factor frequently encountered in the healthcare setting is anxiety. This is 'vague persistent feeling of impending doom' (Arnold and Underman Boggs, 2011: 153). Often hospital routines and procedures that are straightforward to you as a nurse may be a source of anxiety for patients. This anxiety can be reduced through:

- active listening,
- honesty,
- explanation of procedures,
- acting calm and unhurried,
- providing all information about results, restrictions, treatments,
- provide structure,
- explore reasons,
- play therapy, drawing,
- therapeutic intervention (for example, massage),
- breathing and relaxation exercises, and
- guided imagery.

Patient-centred communication

Patient-centred care is a concept with which nurses are familiar because it is often referred to in nurse education and nursing theory as the context in which nurses should plan, organize and provide patient care. Patient-centred communication is defined as 'communication that invites and encourages the patient to participate and negotiate in decision-making regarding their own care' (Langwitz et al. 1998: 230). While participation and negotiation are regarded as key elements in patient-centred communication, it could be argued that the use of the term 'invites' implies that the balance of power and control in this relationship lies with the nurse. However, for communication to be patient-centred, power and control need to be shared equally between the nurse and the patient. This can be a challenge for nurses because as mentioned in relation to Buber's I-Thou theory if nurses are socialized by the culture and organization of nurse education and healthcare management into a task-centred approach to patient care. This means that nurses adopt a communication style that focuses on the completion of tasks relating to patients rather than communicating with the patient as a person with their own individual needs.

Rogers' (1961) views certain qualities in a nurse, such as, warmth, genuineness and empathy as a prerequisite for communication to be patient-centred. This implies that it is not enough to invite or encourage a patient to participate and negotiate in planning their own care, as this will only be successful if it is done within the context of warmth, genuineness and empathy. Buber's I-Thou theory that states that mutual respect as individuals, equal commitment and responsibility are essential ingredients in a relationship is communicated in the nurse–patient relationship through warmth, genuineness and empathy. The nurse will know by the feedback from the patient whether or not they perceive the nurse to have a genuine concern for them as an individual. They will respond by smiling and telling the nurse about themselves.

A key point in the successful development of a patient-centred relationship is the value that nurses place on this relationship. A nurse although working within a patient-centred system of patient care, such as team nursing, may have the I-It view of patients and view the planning and organization of patient care as a series of tasks to be completed within the duration of a working day. These tasks may be completed efficiently and competently. However, this approach can leave the patient feeling very detached and even lonely. A narrative from a study by McCabe (2004) on nurse–patient communication from a patient's perspective demonstrates this, 'the only time they'd sit down was when they were taking your blood pressure ... they'd sit there for a few minutes and then move on to the next patient'. When asked if the nurses spoke when they sat down, this participant said 'very little, I think that's the slackest part but as I said, they can't be sitting down talking with patients – I'd say they'd be neglecting their own work then' (McCabe 2004). This patient does not regard himself as being connected with the work of the nurse, the relationship appears very detached and the patient very isolated. The nurse on the other hand feels satisfied or relieved that she is getting through her workload and appears to be competent and efficient. In relation to Freud's view on counter-transference, it is only by bringing our communication behaviours into our awareness that we can begin to use responses that are patient-centred rather than responses based on personal feelings and experiences and needs.

Maslow's (1954) hierarchy of needs advocates the recognition of the person as a 'whole' with specific needs, starting with physiological needs (food, water, sleep, warmth) as the foundations for achieving other needs, such as, safety, the need to belong, the need for a positive self-esteem and finally the need for self-actualization. This provides a framework for nurses in prioritizing the needs of a patient however, often in nursing we talk about the physical and psychological needs of patients as almost separate parts of the person but as the following narrative from McCabe's (2004) study demonstrates, they are inextricably linked, 'I didn't have a shower for the first two days, it just would have taken somebody sensitive enough to understand... I mean you can imagine what you feel like when you can't even wash yourself' (McCabe 2004). The lack of attention to the physical needs of this patient left her feeling frustrated and unable to trust the nurses.

Interestingly this study shows that patients watch nurses at work very closely, not only to determine if they are nice people and trustworthy but also to see if they are competent at nursing skills, using equipment and anticipating their needs (McCabe 2004). For patients, patient-centred care relates to the ability to trust nurses to both anticipate their care needs and provide care competently using the necessary equipment and skills (McCabe 2004). This is another example of how the physical care of a patient impacts on how patients perceive communication in the healthcare context. If they do not feel that the nurse is a safe practitioner they will not trust them and this will impact negatively on the development of the nurse–patient relationship regardless of the communication approach used by the nurse.

By attending to and anticipating the physical needs of a patient, nurses are also attending to their psychological needs but in order for this to be patient-centred it requires that the patient perceives the nurse to be warm, genuine and empathetic. If this does not happen then the patient will not trust the nurse and may appear withdrawn or unfriendly from the nurse's perspective whereas they may just be lonely and feeling isolated. When a patient feels this way, it is very difficult for a nurse to establish a positive relationship. As 'The Comforting Interaction-Relationship Model' (Morse et al. 1997) in Chapter 1 suggests the duration of a relationship is not a factor in whether it is patient-centred or not. It is to do with whether the nurse views the patient in a holistic way as a unique individual and can communicate in a warm, genuine and empathetic manner in meeting the needs of the patient.

If therapeutic communication is about making a patient feel relaxed and secure then another essential ingredient in establishing a therapeutic relationship is patient-centred communication. Patient-centred communication involves:

- active listening and active listening responses;
- building rapport, including initial presentation;
- observation; and
- asking open questions, focused questions and specific closed questions (Arnold and Underman Boggs 2011)

This makes patients feel that they are respected as individuals and that nurses have a genuine concern for their well-being and that they, the patient, have control over the care they receive. The absence of a patient-centred approach to communication will inhibit the development of a therapeutic nurse–patient relationship.

Thus the key characteristics of therapeutic nurse–patient communication include:

- appearance of caring,
- openness,
- warmth,
- genuineness,
- empathy, and
- purpose.

You will see that many of these resonate with Carl Rogers work discussed earlier and with Maslow's self-actualization.

McCormack and McCance (2006) outlined elements that are required for patient-centred care to take place:

1. *Prerequisites* – these are attributes of the nurse such as being competent, having developed interpersonal skills, having job commitment, being self-aware and showing clarity of beliefs and values.

2. *The care environment* – this focuses on the environment within which care is delivered. Patient-centred environments are those where staff: adopt a person-centred approach, take time to understand patients as individuals, and take great effort to include patients in care (Wheeler 2010). It also requires:

   o an appropriate staffing skill mix,
   o systems that facilitate shared decision making,
   o effective staff relationships,
   o supportive organizational systems,
   o the sharing of power,
   o the potential for innovation and risk-taking, and
   o strong nursing leadership.

3. *Person-centred processes* – for patient-centredness to occur processes that need to be present include:

   o working with patient's beliefs and values,
   o engagement,
   o having a sympathetic presence,
   o sharing,
   o involving patients in decision making, and
   o providing for patients' physical needs.

   Interestingly while sympathy is discussed infrequently in nursing patients McCabe's (2004) identified this as a component of effective nurse–patient relationships. Similarly a study by Coyle and Williams (2001) identified that staff needed to be more sensitive to patient illness and treatment effects and be more approachable thus, patient-centred care is important to patients.

4. *Person-centred outcomes* – these relate to evidence that patient-centred care has taken place and include:

   o patient satisfaction with care,
   o patient and family involvement with care, and
   o patient/family's feeling of well-being

Developing awareness of one's own communication behaviour

From the nurses' perspective it is helpful to use Maslow's hierarchy of needs to consider the extent to which self-actualization has been achieved. The characteristics of self-actualization are as follows:

- genuineness,
- integrity,
- responsibility,
- a passion for living,
- an ability to get along with others,
- a high sense of personal worth,
- see life situations as opportunities not threats,
- making most of experiences, and
- an acceptance of self and others.

As you can see a person who has achieved this level of development has a high sense of self-worth and is accepting of others, thus situations of counter transference described above are less likely to occur. Genuineness, integrity and responsibility are also essential skills for nurses. Achieving self-actualization can be developed through improving self-awareness.

Exercise

Consider the components of self-actualization above.
Write down on a scale of 1 to 5 how you see yourself performing in each of these components.
Now ask a friend to do the same, and compare the results.

This exercise will have given you some idea of your strengths in this area and areas you need to develop. This increasing self-awareness of your communication skills is very important in nursing as communicating with patients and families is not just about getting along with them, a nurse needs to have very highly-developed sense of self and a very mature outlook toward others. Developing an awareness of how to change your communication behaviour is also important.

Developing awareness of, and changing, communication behaviour

The process of becoming aware of how we communicate as individuals is a challenging process. It requires nurses to discuss, with other nursing colleagues, the interactions between themselves and their patients. It may be more comfortable initially to discuss issues with someone unrelated to work. You might find it easier to do this on a one-to-one basis initially but as you become better at talking about how you communicate and contributed (good and bad) to interactions with patients it may be more beneficial to do this with a group of work colleagues that you trust and regard as role models.

The focus of these discussions should be to determine whether the interaction was patient-centred. If as a group it is agreed that this was not patient-centred it is essential to determine why it was not and what factors prevented this from happening. Before ending the discussion it is imperative for the development of patient-centred communication that the group decide what specific communication behaviours would have facilitated patient-centred communication in this interaction. It is these interactions that need to be remembered and used consciously in future interactions with patients.

Therapeutic communication

Knowledge of how human beings behave and what motivates human behaviour is important for providing nurses and other healthcare professionals with an understanding of why therapeutic communication is important when caring for people and will also help in using therapeutic skills more effectively. The term therapeutic has connotations of healing or towards improving health and is a term associated primarily with counselling or psychotherapy. Therapeutic communication is a term that is used widely in nursing and in relation to counselling and psychotherapy. In order to provide clarity, the meaning of the term in both contexts will be explored. In counselling and psychotherapy the concept of therapeutic communication requires the presence of a person (counsellor or psychotherapist) who is perceived as having specialist knowledge, experience and communication skills. The sole purpose of therapeutic communication in this context is to encourage and facilitate the development of communication skills in those with immature or disturbed behaviour. This takes place in the context of a professional relationship in which the counsellor or therapist provides specific time, attention and venue for the client or patient.

However since Peplau's (1952) work, nurse theorists and nurse educators have referred to the importance of nurses developing a therapeutic relationship with patients. Today's nursing regulatory bodies confirm the requirement of establishing and maintaining caring therapeutic interpersonal relationships with individuals/clients/groups/communities. (An Bord Altranais 2005). The aim of nurses using therapeutic communication skills is not to treat or cure a disease or disorder rather it is to provide a sense of well-being for patients by making them feel relaxed and secure. Arnold and Underman Boggs (2011: 175) described therapeutic communication as 'an interactive dynamic process entered into by nurse and client for the purpose of achieving health-related goals'. Therapeutic communication is a 'goal-directed' form of communication used in healthcare to achieve goals that 'promote client health and wellbeing' (Arnold and Underman Boggs 2011: 15). Importantly this is different from the 'social chit chat' that is often relied upon to fill the void of communication (Arnold and Underman Boggs 2011: 105). Within the context of nursing therapeutic communication involves:

- exchanging information with patients;
- finding out what they know about their condition, and what l they need to know;
- planning treatment approaches;
- reaching consensus about treatment decisions;
- providing treatment and interventions; and

- evaluating treatment outcomes. (Arnold and Underman Boggs 2011).

All of these above help establish rapport and trust between nurse and patient. These are essential ingredients for the development of a positive nurse–patient relationship. Therapeutic communication results in a focused and purposeful relationship established by the nurse in order to assess, plan, implement and evaluate the care needed by a patient. It is:

- a healing relationship;
- between nurse and patient;
- needs based;
- goal driven: promotion of patients health and being; and
- is termed a therapeutic, or helping relationship. (Arnold and Underman Boggs 2011)

The duration of the relationship is not a factor in establishing a therapeutic nurse–patient relationship. What is required is that the nurse is competent in the nursing skills required to deliver care safely. A therapeutic relationship differs from a social relationship because:

- the nurse takes responsibility for the relationship;
- it is health-goal oriented and purposeful;
- the relationship usually ceases when goal achieved;
- it is usually limited in its choice of personnel; and
- it requires limited self-disclosure by the nurse. (Arnold and Underman Boggs, 2011)

Exercise

Consider the case of Mr. Aadesh Chandak who is a 56-year-old gentleman who has recently undergone a coronary angioplasty.

Although you have almost completed your nurse education programme, you are new to the ward, and have not nursed on a cardiac ward for some time. During the course of the morning you encounter Mr. Chandak:

> *Nurse:* Did you enjoy the match last night Aadesh?
> *Another patient on the ward:* Great score for Hamilton eh?
>   That knocked QPR right out of the league.
> *Mr. Chandak:* Hmmm.
> *Nurse:* Would you believe I had free tickets but couldn't go
>   cause of my late shift.
> *Mr. Chandak:* Well you're lucky to have a job aren't you.
>
> Afterwards you mention to your mentor that while you
> were getting along great with the other patients, Mr.
> Chandak was a bit gruff with you. She informs you that he
> has been a little withdrawn and difficult, and you aim to
> say little to him from now on.
>
> What do you think went wrong?
> How could the communication be improved

Replacing this conversation with therapeutic communication would first involve you getting to know Mr. Chandak's condition much better. Even though you are new to the cardiac ward it is important to understand the individual needs of patients and their health goals. This is fundamental to the therapeutic relationship. You could find out this information by looking through patient charts, care pathways or plans and/or by speaking with your mentor. Once you have a better understanding of his plan of care and information needs your conversation may begin with any of the following:

1. *Nurse*: Mr. Chandak how are you feeling today?
2. *Nurse*: Mr. Chandak I believe that you are meeting with the Cardiac Rehabilitation Nurse today is there anything you would like to know about the visit?
3. *Nurse*: Mr. Chandak I believe that you going home tomorrow, is there any information that you need?
4. *Nurse*: Mr. Chandak what do you know about your reason for admission to hospital?
5. *Nurse*: Mr. Chandak can you tell me about your hospital experience?

These are just examples, but give you an idea about how simple communication can be transformed from chit chat (that may not be appropriate to all patients, or desired by all) to therapeutic communication. Therapeutic communication obviously requires a competence in the field under discussion, however, if you look at the examples above you will see that any questions arising from your questions may be passed onto a more senior nurse if necessary.

The example above demonstrates how social chit chat may not always be appropriate, although a certain level of this conversation, known as 'phatic' communication, is acceptable depending on the circumstances (Morrissey and Callaghan 2011). It is important to remember that this social chit chat complies with cultural norms. It is all too common for nurses to consider their local parlance (and required responses) as generalizable across all cultures, which is not always the case (Burnard and Gill 2009). However, it is important to realize that ultimately communication in nursing needs to be therapeutic and do people good rather than harm, so as nurse you should always be mindful and aware of both your communication and its effect.

In the example above, discussing sport, however well intended may not have been patient centred in this case possibly as the patient had no interest in sport, or was not too concerned about it at this time. Coyle and Williams (2001) study of 97 patients from general wards found that patients required:

- more involvement in care,
- more information,
- increased sensitivity by staff to the impact of their illness and treatment on their life, and
- increased approachability of staff.

Coyle and Williams also recommended 'asking patients regularly about their feelings and views and encouraging them to ask questions ... to clarify the extent to which they what to be involved [in their care]' (2001: 456).

Similarly Wheeler's (2010: 19) interviews with 36 staff caring for older people with dementia found important elements of communication involved the nurses 'talking while doing' , involving the family and helping the older person to reminisce. One effective strategy was '[while dressing them] picking up a picture and saying, "Oh, who's this?" And talking about that person' (Wheeler's 2010: 19). Although on the surface this phatic communication may seem superficial it was beneficial to patients because it involved the patient (was patient centred) and made the patient and family feel good (therapeutic). Wheeler's (2010) study also found that good communication occurred in facilities where staff adopted a person-centred approach, took time to understand patients as individuals and made a great effort to include patients in care.

However Suikkala et al. (2009) found that nursing students' relationships with patients could be categorized as:

- mechanistic,
- authoritative, or
- facilitative.

Mechanistic (Suikkala et al. 2009) communication:

- is focused on student learning,
- is externally directed (by nurse)
- is where student and patient don't know each other,
- focuses on technical performance,
- has little discussion and
- involves the student as observer.

Authoritative (Suikkala et al. 2009) communication:

- is focused on assumptions of what is best for the patient,
- includes decisions taken by the student,
- is where the student knows the patient and condition;
- is where conversation care related,
- provides daily care and
- involves patients asking for advice.

Facilitative (Suikkala et al. 2009) communication:

- focuses on the common good of both the student and the patient,
- is directed by patient wishes
- is where student and patient know each other personally,

- is where the student listens
- focuses on patient's emotions
- involves confidential matters
- is where the student acts as the patient's advocate
- requires the student to encourage patient, and
- the patient gives advice.

Exercise

Consider the communication with Mr. Chandak above. Would you consider this communication to be mechanistic, authoritative or facilitative? Write a couple of lines Consider ways the communication with Mr. Chandak may be improved – write 2 to 3 lines.

Rather than measuring the success of your communications based on the head nodding and smiling of patients (which could be due to politeness and desire to please), consider other ways of examining the effectiveness of your communications. As described above the effectiveness of patient-centred communication needs to be evaluated in order for patient-centred care to have been truly said to occur (McCormack and McCance 2006). You may self-reflect on the extent to which you were patient-centred or facilitative (as in the last exercise) or there may be opportunities for you to be observed in practice, perhaps providing patient education with your mentor present. Afterwards you could seek advice and feedback about your communication skills. Remember it is important that you actively seek out and ask for these opportunities for teaching and learning. A mentor may not specifically choose to monitor your communication in this way, but you might choose to ask for this close scrutiny to build on and improve your communication skills. While constructive feedback can sometimes be difficult to take (we all like to think we are good communicators) you have to keep in mind the following:

- Improvement is always possible.
- Good communication provides good patient care.

- Patients and families frequently complain about communication in the healthcare setting, so you need to be sure that you are doing your very best.
- It is not always possible for us to perceive or judge our own communication skills, so having others do so provides valuable information.
- Developing effective and appropriate interpersonal skills can be a real challenge for some students – using every opportunity to improve is important.

Other ways that you might learn about ways to communicate effectively are by examining evidence. You might ask your mentor for advice about good communication, for example:

- How do you find it best to talk to patients when they are first back from surgery?
- From your experience on this ward what is the best way to ......?
- This is my first time on an oncology ward can you advise me about......?

It is also important to read back through your notes from classes that you may have attended and to read books and articles on the subject of communication. All too often when immersed in the practical elements of the course there is a temptation to put aside the books and learn on the job. However, you are required to be a knowledgeable doer, so we would advise revising your theoretical work in relation to communication and examine ways that you can apply it to practice. The ward or hospital may have also have audit data that you might be permitted to look at, or complaints reports, that while not about you personally may give an indication of the types of communications liked or disliked by patients and their families. Experiences of poor communication in the healthcare setting is a major element of patient and family complaint, and may feature on audit or evaluation forms, so it is worth finding out patient/family experiences for yourself.

Exploring the literature can also improve your understanding and awareness. Using a database such as CINAHL you could search using key terms such as communication, interpersonal, relationship, information and angioplasty (in the case described earlier) to identify studies that have explored this topic. Qualitative studies, such as McCabe's (2004), that write of experiences of speaking directly with patients about communication experiences can be particularly enlightening, although the particular local context of these studies needs to be borne in mind, as they are not deemed scientific fact.

For undergraduate nursing students and newly qualified nurses, therapeutic patient-centred communication may be perceived as a complex and time-consuming process. Within the modern healthcare structure the time a patient spends in hospital is often very short. Day surgery facilities are increasingly common. Although patients' needs may vary between being complex or emotionally difficult to deal with or very straightforward, the majority wants the best treatment possible, delivered in a context that is helpful, positive and meets their specific needs. Even in emergency departments where nurse–patient relationships are of very short duration and often very intense, the most effective therapeutic communication skills are smiling, some eye contact, a calm steady tone of voice and open, honest communication. However, what is required is that nurses are aware of their own communication abilities and limitations and when patients need specialized therapeutic communication, nurses will discuss this with the patient and their doctor. As discussed previously the communication skills required to be therapeutic are no different to those used by people in ordinary everyday situations, however, the focus is at all times on the patient and on the goals of care. Key nurse behaviours include: competence in the field; genuineness; warmth; sympathy/sensitivity; openness; and verbal and non-verbal communication skills such as, listening, questioning and observation. Observation will be discussed in detail in the next chapter. The organization also plays a role in effective communication and both systems and processes need to be in place to support patient centred therapeutic communication.

Key points

▶ Psychological theories are useful in explaining the concept of patient-centredness.

▶ Theories by psychologists such as, Maslow (1954), Rogers (1961) and Freud can help nurses understand and become aware of their own behaviour and that of others.

▶ The development of a positive patient-centred relationship depends largely on the values held by nurses in relation to their role as nurses in the provision of holistic and individualized care.

▶ Therapeutic communication is focused and purposeful and makes patients feel relaxed and secure.

▶ Nurses need to be caring, open, warm, genuine, empathic and purposeful in order to communicate therapeutically.

PART II

The Communication Process in Nursing

4 Communication Skills

Introduction

Communication skills are often classified as verbal and non-verbal with verbal, or the spoken word being regarded as a key component in delivering a message. However, according to Argyle et al. (1970) in an interaction words make up 7 per cent of a message, tone, tempo and syntax make up 38 per cent and body language makes up 55 per cent. This implies that although sometimes it is essential to use appropriate words when sending a message the factors mentioned are a great deal more important than the words used.

> *Example*
> When was the last time you were aware of giving someone a dirty look?
> Why did you give the dirty look?
> How did people respond to you?

This is an example of negative communication (can be conscious or unconscious behaviour) and highlights that just because we do not speak does not mean that we are not communicating.

The skills that are generally described as basic communication skills include listening, questioning, body language and paralinguistics. However, it is probably more accurate to say that these communication skills and others that we will look at in this chapter are best defined as *core* communication skills rather than basic. *Core* communication skills are skills that most human beings have but individuals use these skills in various ways across many different contexts and with different levels of ability. The term *basic* implies skills that are simple and easy to achieve and in a way this term is appropriate because most of us are born with the ability to listen, ask questions and use our bodies to communicate. The natural ease with which most humans develop communication skills from birth may explain why we perceive these skills as basic and even common sense. We, therefore, undervalue their role as core communication skills because they form all or parts of all communication.

The perception of listening, questioning, body language and paralinguistics as basic communication skills can also be the reason why communication between people is sometimes very effective and positive and other times, it is ineffective, difficult and negative. As communication is perceived as a natural phenomenon, people generally do not think about how they communicate with others and feel that the way they communicate is beyond their control. Personality is often linked to the way a person communicates. It is perceived as a permanent aspect of our character and therefore, cannot be changed. Developing your communication skills is not about changing your personality; it is about developing and adapting your behaviour and responses in interactions with others in order to communicate positively and effectively with others.

In Chapter 1 you were asked to think about what communication is. You may have found this difficult because you do not generally think about communication and probably almost never discuss your communication skills with another person. We are generally much better at critically examining other people's communication skills than our own! However, communication is a complex process that requires the use of core communication skills within many interactions throughout a day. The appropriate and effective use of these skills requires practice. This can be a challenge initially because we so rarely think consciously about how we communicate; therefore, practicing these skills seems difficult and false. Developing effective communication skills is a similar process to acting. You learn your lines and you decide how your character should behave when delivering the lines. Students often tell us that if learning to communicate well requires acting then it is false and they are not being honest. When learning to communicate, the purpose of this acting is not to be false or dishonest with others, it is to learn about and practice using specific communication skills appropriately and effectively in many different contexts. Like any skill, for example, playing a musical instrument, to do it well, you need to practice regularly and you get better every time you practice. Eventually you will be able to play a piece of music without thinking about it but you will not succeed unless you want to learn how to play the instrument. The same goes for learning to communicate well, you will not succeed unless you are prepared to examine you current communication behaviour and consciously learn and practice new communication skills and develop and focus the skills that you already have.

Exercise

Ask a person who knows you well, for example, a family member, partner or friend, to tell you what they think of your communication skills. You may have to tell them what you mean by communication because, remember like most people, they do not generally think about what communication is and may not know what information you are looking for. You might find it useful to ask them to rate your skills from 0–100 but they will need to explain their answer!

Most of us think we are better communicators than we really are so be prepared for the answer!

Communication is an integral part of nursing and therefore needs to be considered carefully and addressed both on a personal and professional basis by all nursing students. In order to use communication skills in a patient-centred way, nurses need not only to learn about and practice communication skills, they also need to have certain professional characteristics. These include genuineness, warmth and the ability to be empathetic. These characteristics come naturally to some people but others have to work at developing these characteristics by being non-judgmental towards patients, accepting patients as unique individuals and developing awareness of their own communication ability and work at addressing deficits.

Establishing rapport

Communication skills, such as, listening, questioning, touch, paraphrasing and body language are used specifically by nurses in developing a trusting relationship or what is often referred to as *rapport* with patients. This is the foundation stone of a positive nurse–patient relationship and is worth spending time on when you meet a patient for the first time. First impressions count so it is important to introduce yourself, smile, lean towards the patient, look directly at them and begin the interaction with an open ended question such as, 'how are you today?'. These communication behaviours convey warmth and genuineness to patients (Fleischer et al. 2009; Williams 2001).

Appearances also matter. Patients observe the physical appearance of the nurse, for example, how she wears her uniform and the expression on her face and based on their own personal values and beliefs they will decide if a nurse looks like a *good* person and, therefore, trustworthy (McCabe 2010). This only takes a few seconds and influences the patient's initial response; therefore, the nurse needs to be aware of the message that her appearance is sending to patients. If a nurse looks untidy she may be perceived as disinterested, lazy and even incompetent even if this is not the case. Awareness of the non-verbal messages we send to others is essential, as it will often provide an explanation as to why people respond to us the way they do.

Listening

Listening is one of the most important of the non-verbal communication skills and its value is often underestimated. Hearing what another person is saying to us is just a small part of listening, remember, non-verbal communication makes up most of an interaction. Furthermore, we may hear what somebody is saying to us but that doesn't mean that we are actively listening. When you actively listen to another person it means that you are demonstrating your commitment to them as a unique individual, you want to help or comfort them, you want to understand them and you want to learn something or you may just want to enjoy their company. Active listening requires that you give the other person your complete attention. This is conveyed primarily through the use of body language with minimal verbal interaction. 'You must be silent if you wish to listen to another, to listen with openness. This involves silencing not only your mouth but also your mind' (Perry 1996: 9). Gibbons (1993) suggested that nurses find it difficult to be silent because of their work is so action oriented. This does not bode well for nurses' ability to actively listen to their patients. Silence is not an unresponsive communication. It is a skill, which, if used appropriately, gives patients a sense of time to think and talk. It also gives time to the nurse to respond in an appropriate and patient-centred way. The following steps may help you to develop your active listening skills:

- When the other person speaks to you, look at them with an open and interested expression on your face. This may be frustrating if you are busy and do not feel like it. It requires a conscious effort on your part to stop thinking about what you were doing and stop wondering when you will get back to it.
- Allow the person to speak without interrupting them and as they speak take note of how they are speaking and the body language they use. Awareness of this will provide you with more information about what they are feeling and what they are trying to say even though the words they use may not reflect this. Use some eye contact and prompts such as nodding your head to encourage them to speak freely and develop their thoughts.
- When you respond make sure that you reflect their feelings and that your facial expression and tone are appropriate and match what you are trying to say. You may need to clarify what they have said by asking questions and summarizing what they said. This does not send the message that you were not listening to instead it demonstrates that you are interested in ensuring that you got the message correctly and you are trying to fully understand what they are saying.

● Observe the feedback that you receive from the other person. If they seem happy with what you said or try to continue the conversation then you can be sure that you have interpreted their words and body language correctly.

Feedback and clarification are two key characteristics of active listening. A third is paraphrasing (DeVito 2011). Paraphrasing is repeating something that someone else said in your own words. In order to repeat what you have just heard you need to listen carefully. This demonstrates to others that you have been listening; therefore, you are interested in what they are saying. Paraphrasing prevents misunderstanding and misinterpretation of information and encourages communication that is open. In other words, you are so intent on listening to another person that you forget to be judgmental or you do not feel that you need to interrupt to say what you want to say.

Exercise

Ask a friend or partner to tell you how their day went at work in detail. When they have finished repeat what they told you in your own words. Don't be too surprised at what you leave out or get confused! If you get it right and leave nothing out, think about whether you listened differently to the way you normally listen to patients – be honest with yourself!

This type of communication can also be described as genuine behaviour. It is open, non-judgmental and your body language is congruent with the words that you use. In nursing active listening is often regarded by nurses as a time-consuming process. This is not the case and if a nurse is genuinely interested in a patient and what they have to say, active listening can be used effectively in even the briefest and transient of encounters. However, instead of actively listening to patients, nurses can appear to be listening to patients in that they respond to what the patient says in a friendly and appropriate manner but they do not stop what they are doing or look directly at the patient when they respond. They may continue to adjust the intravenous line beside the patient or document the patient's vital signs or fluid intake without ever looking directly at them. This is false listening and gives the patient the message that the nurse is too busy to talk to them so they refrain from asking too many questions or discussing their care.

Scenario 1

A patient is lying in bed at 10 a.m. and would like to have a shower. However, an intravenous infusion is in progress and there is still a small amount of fluid remaining. The alarm sounds on the infusion pump so the patient rings the nurse call bell to get a nurse's attention. A few minutes later a nurse enters the room and turns off the alarm. She says in a friendly voice 'I'll be back in a few minutes to deal with that for you' and leaves quickly. The patient waits for her return but after 20 minutes assumes that the nurse has forgotten because she is so busy. The alarm on the infusion pump sounds again so the patient rings the nurse call bell once more. The same nurse returns and as responds to the alarm she says in a friendly and apologetic voice ' I am sorry about earlier on, I got caught up doing something and didn't get back to you, I'll just go and finish what I was doing and come straight back'. The patient says 'that's fine nurse and maybe you could help me to the shower then?' as the nurse leaves the room. 'Of course' the nurse says and the patient waits again for her to return.

Scenario 2

A patient is lying in bed at 10 a.m. and would like to have a shower. However, an intravenous infusion is in progress. The alarm sounds on the infusion pump so the patient rings the nurse call bell to get a nurse's attention. A few minutes later a nurse enters the room. She smiles at the patient and turns off the alarm. She looks at the patient and says, 'I'll be back in ten minutes to deal with that for you'. The patient says, 'that's great and maybe you could assist me with a shower then'. 'Yes certainly and perhaps after the shower you might like me to escort you on a walk down the corridor?' The patient nods their head and smiles in agreement and starts go gather things from their locker for the shower. The nurse returns ten minutes later as arranged.

The nurse in both of these scenarios was friendly and responded to the call bell quickly. However, in Scenario 1, the patient was left feeling let down and possibly frustrated by the nurse because although friendly the nurse did not return when she said she would and she did not look directly at the patient throughout the interaction. This is an example of false listening and can be perceived by the patient as detachment or disinterest. The patient will find it difficult to trust this nurse and will probably stop the next nurse that comes into the room and ask her to help them have a shower. The nurse in the second scenario was also friendly but she also looked directly at the patient, smiled and in a very informal way, negotiated a short-term plan of care that met both their needs. This patient trusted the nurse because they knew they would obtain assistance with the shower and be able to take a walk when the nurse returned. This is an example of active listening that is patient-centred communication. As a student or junior staff nurse, you might have experienced similar feelings when trying to get the attention of a senior staff member. You ask a question once and if you don't get a response that you trust, you are less likely to approach that person again!

Exercise

Have you ever been in a supermarket and gone through the checkout, paid for your groceries and said goodbye and thanked the person at the checkout without looking directly at them? If you can't remember or don't know, next time you go in make a conscious effort to look at the person when you speak to them. If it feels odd, then you know that not looking directly at them is your normal behaviour. After this exercise think about how the person at the checkout responded when you looked directly at them and how this made you feel.

Exercise

Imagine being in a restaurant or a pub chatting to a friend. You have your back to the door and your friend is facing the door. You are both having a good time chatting but every now and then your friend looks over your shoulder towards the door. This is irritating and you start looking in the same direction and ask her what she's looking at. 'Nothing' she answers and continues talking. How does this make you feel?

Now think of a person that you do not normally pay much attention to or just pretend to listen to because you do not like them and find them boring. Next time you meet them try active listening and afterwards think about how it changed the pattern of the type of interactions you previously had with that person. You may not feel any different about the other person but you both will probably have had a much more positive interaction.

Touch

Physical touches can a very powerful communication strategy when helping patients meet their physical needs and actively listening to another person.

- Touch can be empathetic by demonstrating understanding and support and can consequently alleviate patient anxiety and worry.
- Touch can provide comfort and security for patients who are distressed or perhaps scared about their illness.
- Touch can add meaning or emphasis to the spoken word.

Touch can be classified as instrumental, expressive or demonstration (Roberts and Bucksey 2007). Instrumental touch is the physical touch required to complete a task related to the physical needs of a patient. This is also referred to as functional touch. Expressive touch is regarded as spontaneous and connecting with the patient as an individual on an emotional and possibly spiritual level. Demonstration touch is primarily associated with educating patients about how to self-manage (Roberts and Bucksey 2007). However, the findings from research on the use of physical touch in nursing vary widely. This may be because the experience of touch for individuals is so subjective and contextually driven that it is extremely difficult to identify general experiences. In conjunction with other communication behaviours such as eye contact, smiling and speech, touch can have a calming and comforting effect on patients. However, not all touch will have this affect and it is important for nurses to use touch in situations/interactions in which it is appropriate and also to ensure that the manner in which they use touch is appropriate. The issue for nurses is how to know if a patient wants or is responding positively to touch. It is, therefore, important to observe the feedback from the patient. If they withdraw from a touch to the arm or shoulder then they are probably uncomfortable or may not trust the nurse. Respect for patients' personal and cultural difference will help prevent situations that are inappropriate and/or uncomfortable for both the nurse and the patient. Active listening is also a key element in accurately identifying if touch is appropriate or not.

Example
Nurse: Let me help you change those pyjamas
Patient: Thanks, oooh, your hands are cold (with a laugh)
Nurse: Yes, everyone tells me that, but you know what they say? Cold hands – Warm heart (laughing)

This exchange is open and friendly but the nurse has not listened to what the patient was saying. The nurse should have responded by apologizing and then running her hands under warm water to warm them up. Has anyone ever put a cold hand on you? You respond very quickly and move out of their reach! Well that's how a patient wants to react but can't because they need the nurse's help.

The way in which nurses use touch is influenced by their age, sex, culture, education level, and the part of the body to be touched so even if you are not the type of person that generally uses expressive touch that does not mean that you do not communicate a message to patients when you touch them. Instrumental touch can also be calming and comforting for patients. This is because patients will feel the intention of your touch in the way that you deliver physical care. If your hands are warm and your touch is relaxed and smooth, with eye contact and appropriate verbal cues, this will transmit a positive feeling to patients. Any combination of jerky movements along with cold hands and a 'busy' persona will transmit a more negative feeling to patients.

Exercise

Try this with a friend or work colleague
First shake hands and as you do take note of how their skin feels against yours. Is it warm, hot, cold, cool, smooth, rough, sweaty, firm grip or weak grip? Then ask the other person to tell you how your hand felt to them.
   The purpose of this exercise is to develop awareness of the experience of touch for you and patients and how it can influence responses in an interaction.

Questioning

Questioning is another core communication skill that we use to meet many communication goals. These include:

- Starting a conversation or keeping a conversation going.
- Gain information about others – this can be broad or specific.
- Increase our knowledge.
- Encourage participation and involvement in group discussions.
- Encourage others to reflect, evaluate and be critical.
- Determine level of knowledge in others.
- Control conversations.

The achievement of any of these goals requires the use of one or more types of questions. Questions can be classified as open, closed and circular questions and are classified according to the amount of information required in response to the question.

Types of questions

Open questions are questions that give the respondent the opportunity to give as much or as little information as they wish when responding to a question. Asking open questions in an atmosphere that is relaxed and comfortable for patients encourages them to talk freely and for longer periods. Questions of this type help to build rapport between the nurse and patient. Open questions usually start with 'how', 'what' or 'please tell me about'. Examples of open-ended questions are:

- How are you feeling today?
- What do you think of your new medication?
- Please tell me about the history of your injury.

Open questions can also begin with 'why', for example.

Patient: I didn't go to the doctor until my son called to see me and insisted on taking me.
Nurse: Why didn't you go to the doctor?

This seems like a reasonable question to ask and it is an important one, however the use of the word 'why' can make the patient feel that they did something wrong or that they need to justify their actions. Questions starting with 'why' can also be perceived as aggressive or even judgemental. Another way of asking the same question is:

Patient: I didn't go to the doctor until my son called to see me and insisted on taking me.
Nurse: It sounds like you must have been very unwell.

In nursing, open questions can be used to determine a patients' cognitive ability, recall and their understanding of their care. If a patient is finding it difficult to respond to an open question, prompts, paraphrasing and repeating can be used to encourage the patient to continue talking. When open questions are used at the outset of an interaction, they can provide broad information and the nurse may need to use closed questions to clarify points and elicit specific information.

Closed questions need a limited and specific response. Examples of closed questions include:

- Who is your next of kin?
- What is your name?
- Do you have a pain in your chest?

Closed questions can also be useful in the initial stages of the nurse–patient relationship to get someone talking or 'break the ice'. However, if used excessively closed questions can limit the contribution of the patient to the interaction and result in the nurse controlling the scope and length of the interaction. This type of communication is frequently used in nursing because nurses are busy and usually have a limited amount of time to spend with patients and closed questioning allows nurses to get specific information from patients. However, it does not encourage patients to talk, voice any concerns that they may have or contribute to the conversation generally. It is not patient-centred communication, instead it is task-centred, that is, it allows nurses to interact with patients at a very functional level and with the aim of getting the information they need so that they can proceed with completing any other work that they may have to do.

A combination of open and closed questions that is weighted towards open questions is the best option in nurse–patient communication. Following the patient's primary response to a question, the nurse can ask a probing or clarifying question. This allows nurses to get the specific information that they need and also encourages patients to talk while at the same time demonstrating the nurses' interest in listening to what patients have to say (Hargie 2011). The result is that patients feel valued and cared for as individuals. A rapport develops and this lays the foundation for a positive nurse--patient relationship.

When a nurse asks a patient a question, she needs to listen carefully to the answer the patient gives. The patient may avoid answering the question because the subject matter distresses them or because they did not understand the question. The patient may answer the question but the answer may seem vague or incongruent with the patient's behaviour. The following is an example of how questioning can go wrong:

Nurse: Hi John, has that injection lessened your pain? It should be working by now.

Patient: Eh, yes I think it is (patient appears restless and is finding it difficult to get comfortable)

Nurse: Are you sure John, you don't seem to be comfortable?

Patient: Well actually the injection hasn't made any difference. I'm still in a lot of pain!

The nurse in this scenario asked a very leading question. She implied that the injection should be working and that the patient should be feeling better. The patient, therefore, found it difficult to tell the nurse that the analgesia had not worked and probably felt that if they said nothing and waited a little longer, it would work. In this instance the nurse noticed the patients' incongruent behaviour and realized that he was still in pain. However, leading questions can result in incorrect or misleading responses. The other interesting aspect to this scenario is that even though the nurse asked a leading question, it is apparent that patients often try to give the answer they think the nurse wants to hear. This is another reason why open questions are more patient focused than closed questions.

Sometimes patients do not understand the question because of the terminology used. So simple language is essential and questions that are not lengthy or convoluted.

Example 1
Did you have your first surgery last year when you came in with the perforated ulcer or was that when you needed the laparotomy in 1999?

Example 2
Tell me everything about your illness from day one.

It is also very helpful for patients if nurses tell them why they are asking the questions and what they are going to do with the information.

Example
Hello my name is Jane and I'm going to be admitting you today. I need to ask you some questions that you may have been asked already but I will be recording this information in your nursing notes. This information will be used to identify your needs and help develop a plan of nursing care for you.

The type of question you use should be linked with the ability of the patient to answer. This will be determined by their level of understanding of their illness, level of education and how well or unwell they are. Closed questions are more effective for patients who are unwell or have lower intelligence (Hargie 2011). Open questions on the other hand result in responses that are more accurate, detailed and engaging for the person asking the questions.

Like any other aspect of communication it is important to think about what type of question to use before asking it. This is influenced by the type of information you want, and why you want the information. You may just be asking the patient where they are from because you are interested in them and because you want to get to know them. You also need to choose the language of the question carefully and be very clear in the way that you speak when asking questions. The feedback or response from the patient will tell you whether your question was clear and understood. If you find that the patient does not understand you or misinterprets the question, the problem is more likely to do with how the question was asked than the person misunderstanding or misinterpreting the question.

Information giving

Patients are often reassured when they are given information about their illness, plan of care, the length of time they will be in hospital and how they can cope at home. However, patients can become stressed or even more anxious if they are given too much information over a short period of time. It is always better to ask a patient if they would like more information about something rather than assuming that they do or do not want it. This is particularly important after patients receive a diagnosis of a chronic or life-threatening illness as often they are too upset and need time to consider the implications of their illness. Availability and access to a health professional that can explain the relevant treatment regimens and answer the patient's or their family's questions is essential in the days, weeks and months after diagnosis. This may be face-to-face contact at a clinic, over the telephone, information booklets and/or references to relevant and validated online material.

The type of information a patient needs depends on their level of intelligence, education, previous experience and knowledge of their illness. It can be difficult for a nurse to assess this quickly so a good rule of thumb is always ask the patient to repeat in their own words what you just told them or what they read in the information sheet. This should not be said in a patronizing way and should be preceded by an explanation as to why you are asking them to repeat it. This demonstrates the 'mutuality' of nurse–patient interactions in which the nurse and patient have a responsibility and mutual role to play in the success or otherwise of the interaction (Fleischer et al. 2009).

Written information

Written information should always be provided with verbal information where possible. This is because most patients experience some level of anxiety when in hospital or they may be distracted because most information is given to patients on the day of discharge or in the preceding days. They may receive information about the drugs they will need to take when discharged, outpatient appointments, how to look after their wound or dressing, what they should do and what they shouldn't do – it is hardly surprising that they forget what the nurse has said to them. Furthermore patients are often thinking about how they will cope at home or are busy packing their bags therefore, they miss important information. Preparing patients for discharge well in advance may help patients remember instructions. Giving information to patients when their next-of-kin or relative is present may also be helpful.

The care of an individual who is unwell requires input from many healthcare and non-healthcare professionals. Verbal and written communication is used to ensure that this takes place in an efficient, accurate and safe manner. In nursing, written communication forms the basis of recording information about how nurses assess patients' needs and plan, implement and evaluate their care. Patient's responses to prescribed medication, treatments, investigations and medical/surgical interventions are also documented by nurses in nursing notes. Responses can be recorded using soft (electronic) or hard (paper) methods and are recorded in nursing notes. Other healthcare professionals such as doctors, dieticians, physiotherapists and occupational therapists record information in the relevant notes. It is essential, therefore, that all written records are:

- clear,
- objective,
- relevant,
- written in black (photocopies best), and
- include the date, time and legible signature. (Washer 2009)

Always remember that the way you write about patients and their care reflects directly on your professionalism and that patients, their families, your colleagues and other professionals involved in the care of the patient will read what you write. As a student or newly qualified staff nurse you might find it useful to seek the opinion of the nurse manager on what you write alternatively read the nursing notes of an experienced staff nurse that you feel is a good role model. This will help build you confidence in building what is a key nursing skill but the importance of which is often undervalued.

Paralinguistics

It's not what you say, it's how you say it!

Paralinguistics are non-verbal communications that refer to the tone and pitch of the voice and accent of the speaker and the speed at which they speak. Either on its own or in conjunction with the spoken word paralinguistics is used to express attitudes or emotions. They can also complement or contradict the spoken word. A simple statement can be interpreted in many different ways depending on the tone and pitch of the voice and also the emphasis of the speaker, for example, consider the following statement made by a nurse to a patient:

Wake up, it is time for your medication.

If this is said using a quiet, soft and low tone of voice, the patient will more than likely wake up and take their medication. However, if this is said in a louder, more high-pitched voice, the experience will be quite different for the patient. As you can imagine if you were the patient, it is irritating and demonstrates a lack of consideration on the part of the nurse.

Accents play a key role in establishing a nurse–patient relationship. A query about the accent of the nurse is often a starting point or an icebreaker when a patient meets a nurse for the first time. If the patient or nurse is familiar with the accent it can help them to be more comfortable with each other and help the relationship to develop positively. However, it can also result in labelling and/or prejudice if the patient or nurse has preconceived ideas about the culture or class associated with the accent. If someone speaks with an accent that we find difficult to understand, it causes us to reduce our verbal interaction with that person because asking a person to repeat what they have said more than once can become embarrassing for both people concerned.

It is the way in which paralinguistics are used that ultimately determines how a message is interpreted and responded
to. So if you find yourself walking away from an interaction
saying something like: 'I don't know why he got so annoyed,
I only asked him to turn the television down, it was irritating
everyone!' then think about why you got the response you did.
The reason the man was annoyed was probably to do with the
way he was asked to turn down the television. Most people are
reasonable and if spoken to respectfully can deal with what
they hear very well. It is when the message is delivered in an
authoritative, aggressive or hostile tone that communication
goes wrong and if accompanied with a different tone, the same
message would seem innocuous to most people. The appropriate and effective use of paralinguistics requires awareness of
the use of the tone and pitch of the voice when speaking.
Practice in using a calm and even tone with moderate pitch is
also required. This does not mean that good communication
requires a calm, even and moderate tone all the time but it
does mean that when appropriate, it can be used well, effectively and purposefully.

Empathy

> the ability to perceive and reason as well as the ability to communi-
> cate understanding of the other person's feelings and their attached
> meanings (Reynolds and Scott 2000: 226)

Empathy is a prerequisite for high-quality nursing practice
because it is fundamental to all helping relationships and the
achievement of the goals of clinical nursing (Reynolds and
Scott, 2000; Peplau, 1997; Morse et al. 1992). These goals
include the need to understand patient distress and to provide
supportive interpersonal communication. If nurses fail to
empathize with their patients, then they cannot help them to
understand or cope effectively as individuals with their illness
(Morse et al. 1992; Peplau, 1997; Reynolds and Scott, 2000).
Patients value empathetic communication skills such as understanding and anticipating their needs (McCabe 2004).
However, empathy in nursing is a concept that remains poorly

understood and its impact on patient outcomes is unclear (Kunyk 2001; Reynolds and Scott 2000; Morse et al. 1992). The reason for this could be the traditional association between empathy, in particular 'therapeutic empathy' and the counselling profession. Therapeutic empathy which is 'a learned communication skill comprised primarily of cognitive and behavioural components which is used to convey understanding of the patients reality' is inappropriate because its purpose is to enable the sufferer to gain insight (Morse et al. 1992: 810). However, this conceptualization of empathy is primarily that of professional counsellors but is accepted in nursing without question as the central helping component in nurse–patient interaction. That does not mean that nurses should not use therapeutic empathy. Nurses use aspects of counselling skills in their work on a daily basis but they are not counsellors unless they have a specific counselling qualification and the nurse–patient relationship is recognized formally as a counselling one by the nurse and the patient. The difference between therapeutic communication in nursing and therapeutic communication in counselling and psychotherapy lies not in the communication skills required but in the motivation for using them.

For clarity, the empathy that is suggested for everyday use in nursing is described as basic (Freshwater 2003). This does not mean that it is less valuable or less therapeutic than 'therapeutic empathy'. Basic empathy is patient-centred communication and is essential for helping relationships and for establishing rapport and trust. It is particularly appropriate for nursing because most relationships between nurses and patients are transient and brief but yet may be quite intense in that the nurse is often required to reduce levels of anxiety and deal with emotional aspects of people's lives. Basic empathy is achieved through the use of active listening skills, questioning and touch in a patient-centred way.

The basic requirements of being empathetic are as follows:

- An ability to listen.
- An ability to take on another's term of reference (imagine what it is like to be them).
- An ability to understand and not judge.

- An ability to communicate that understanding. (Wiseman, 1996)

As discussed in Chapter 1, according to Morse et al.'s (1992) model of 'emotional empathy', therapeutic empathetic communication needs to be patient-centred, reflexive and genuine. Specific responses include pity, sympathy, reflexive reassurance and compassion. Responses such as sharing of 'self', reassurance (informing) and therapeutic empathy (learned professional behaviour) are second-level empathetic responses. Non-therapeutic responses include dehumanizing, withdrawing, distancing and labelling.

Morse et al. (1992) proposed that communication responses such as sympathy, pity and commiseration have been devalued and labelled as unhelpful in nursing and healthcare generally. According to Morse et al. (1992) sympathy, which is a first-level empathetic response, is a verbal and non-verbal expression of the nurse's own sorrow or dismay at the patient's situation. When nurses are sympathetic, patients perceive that their feelings of anxiety or distress are justified and value the support from nurses. They find it comforting, reassuring and it can make them feel cared for as an individual. Basic empathetic communication transmits the message of a nurse's understanding and recognition of a patient's situation, it does not mean that nurses are expected to 'fix' or 'solve' all the patient's problems. It is important to note however, that while sympathy, pity and commiseration are valuable empathetic responses, they are part of normal everyday communication and within the context of professional practice; a nurse would be required to provide a greater level of emotional help and support to patients when appropriate. Understanding, recognition and support from the nurse are key factors in helping patients cope with their situation themselves. This narrative from McCabe (2004) illustrates this point:

> I think the reassurance from the nurse with me at the time of my diagnosis made me feel at ease straight away ... She just organized everything and was really relaxed and wasn't watching her watch to see was she running late – she was just awfully concerned and at the same time, very professional. She added the human touch, like as if she knew what it was like in my shoes. (Claire)

This is a second level empathetic response. The nurse has communicated her understanding of Claire's predicament and is reassuring Claire by sharing her 'self'. Morse et al. (1992) describe this type of empathy as 'patient-focused' and results in patients feeling secure and reassured. Nurses need to value this type of communication for the positive influence it can have on patients but use it in a genuine and patient-centred way. At undergraduate level and when newly qualified high level empathetic responses can be difficult and are perhaps not required anyway unless a nurse has the necessary counselling qualifications. What is important is that the nurse is supportive and helpful and can recognize the point when a patient may need to be referred to a counsellor, psychologist or psychiatrist as appropriate.

Key points

▶ Communication can be verbal, non-verbal or written.
▶ Communication skills such as, active listening, questioning, touch, paraphrasing and paralinguistics are core skills that can be developed and used in many different ways in any context.
▶ The development of these core communication skills is essential for therapeutic and patient-centred communication requires motivation and practice on the part of the nurse.
▶ Nurses need to develop awareness about how they use core communication skills and the influence this has on the nurse–patient relationship.
▶ Empathy is an important communication skill for nurses and is an integral skill in developing a therapeutic relationship with patients.
▶ A key aspect of the nurse's role is knowing the limitations of their communication skills and referring the patient to an appropriately skilled person, for example, a counsellor or psychologist if necessary.

5 Barriers to Effective Communication

As highlighted in previous chapters one fundamental value that should underpin your nursing practice is the development of a therapeutic relationship between you and the patient. However, this may seem increasingly difficult as patients stay in hospital less time or your visits in the community are brief. As we discussed in Chapter 3 the routine nature of many care interventions can lead to you feeling under pressure to get the work done. In this sequence of tasks the potential for a therapeutic relationship to occur seems much less. In this context it is accepted that certain barriers exist in the healthcare environment that can affect your ability to make and maintain therapeutic relationships and deliver truly patient-centred care. The purpose of this chapter is to explore these barriers and to look at ways to overcome them.

Barriers to the therapeutic relationship

What are barriers?

Leaving aside the specific healthcare environment for a moment let us consider first the meaning of barriers in communication.

Exercise

Think back to the communication theory in Chapter 1. Outline a simple communication process.

You have probably identified the simplest model of communication, termed the Linear Model (Miller and Nicholson

1976). Understanding communication in this way means that you know that there has to be a sender, and message and a receiver. Now consider the next exercise.

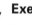

Exercise

Think of things that occur in this process (sender, message and receiver) that prevent the communication being effective? Write two to three lines.

During this exercise above you will probably have noticed that factors in both the sender and receiver can affect communication. In order for a message to be received the sender needs to be capable, verbally or writing (or by other means) of communicating that message, and the receiver needs to be able to both receive, either by hearing or reading (or other means), and interpret the message. Clearly what seems at face value a simple process is actually a complex one.

Exercise

Summarize the broad factors that you think prevent communication being effective in the linear communication process. Write two to three lines.

You will have identified that a range of physical, psychological, environmental issues contribute to the success or otherwise of simple communication. While it is beyond the scope of this book to describe in detail the range of effects, it is important for you to understand first that communication is a complex, rather than a simple, process. Second that the communication interaction needs to be understood in the context of barriers that may exist relating to physical, psychological and environmental issues. Furthermore, as a nurse you need to develop a growing awareness of your own self in the communication process, as your own particular experiences may affect it. Each person is a unique individual with a 'unique interpretation of the world influenced by origin, upbringing and life experience" (Hindle, 2006: 53). Developing an increased self-awareness through reflecting on your communication skills will be discussed in more detail in Chapters 10 and 11. For the moment we will focus on identifying factors within you that can affect the communication.

Personal factors that can affect communication

Aspects present within a person that can distort a message are known as filters (Hindle 2006). Filters can occur due to:

- defence mechanisms,
- attitudes and beliefs,
- values,
- prejudices, and
- perceptual disturbances.

These can adversely affect communication in the healthcare setting. Defence mechanisms are discussed in more detail in Chapter 3. To demonstrate how the other filters operate we ask you to consider the following scenario:

Borkyso Banerek is a 40-year-old gentleman admitted to the hospital for a right knee arthroscopy. Nursing reports on the patient indicate that he is a heavy smoker. The evening before his surgery you notice him take a packet of cigarettes from his locker and put them in his pockets.

Write down your impressions of his actions? What do you think he is going to do? How do you feel about it?

You overhear a nurse say in front of the other patients 'Now Mr. Banerek you know how bad smoking is for you, you shouldn't be smoking, and certainly not here in this ward, you will blow everyone up. Go down to the smoking area if you have to'.

What are your views on this communication interaction? What are your views on Mr. Banerek's smoking? What other ways could stop smoking advice be delivered?

From this scenario above we hope that you will have identified that the nurse's negative attitude towards smoking meant that her interaction with Mr. Banerek was not a positive health enhancing one, but rather a negative interaction that could have left him feeling ashamed and embarrassed. You will see that the nurse did not establish his reasons for his actions, nor his intentions, but simply jumped to conclusions based on personal perceptions/attitudes/beliefs/values/ prejudice. Perceptual distortion was also possible in this case, as the nurse seemed to believe that the patient was going to smoke in the ward, perhaps based on previous experiences, yet there was no specific evidence that pointed to this. This example gives a little insight into how filters can distort communications. Can you imagine the next communication that follows on from this scenario? Write down your ideas.

It is quite possible that this communication may have sparked a negative reaction in Mr. Banerek, leading to conflict. Smoking cessation requires help and support within the healthcare context, and off the cuff remarks like those in the scenario contribute very little to convincing a patient to stop. However, you could find yourself making judgments like this about a patient's behaviour, and commenting upon it, without thinking through what is the best way to deal with it. Behaving assertively and dealing with conflict will be dealt with in more detail in Chapter 8, now we are using this scenario to convince you that communications are influenced by personal factors, therefore the notion of sending a message and receiving it is not as simple as first thought.

These filters that we all possess may form part of our internal frame of reference (Arnold and Underman Boggs 2011), which simply means the standpoint we take, perhaps unknowingly, in response to others. Although we may consider ourselves good communicators, there is a tendency in us all to see the world through our own perspective, without necessarily considering the distinct perspective of the other (Burnard and Gill 2008). It is this perspective that serves as the filter Hindle (2006) describes. Consider the following:

You are with your friend on a train, and you both spot a newspapers headline
'School shock: child kept out of school for six weeks....'
   You can't see the remainder of the story, but your friend whispers to you 'that's dreadful' .
   Write down the thoughts that instantly go through your mind about this possible scenario:
   Consider what you thought of the:

- Parents?
- Child?
- School?
- Reasons for keeping out of school?

You will see from this exercise above that the visions you create that permit you to begin to interpret this communication invariably come from your own experience in life. Your interpretations of parents, children and school are most likely to be based on that which you have seen or experienced. Likewise your understandings of the reasons for keeping a child out of school will be based on these. These interpretations and understandings will also ultimately be influenced by the culture in which you were raised (Burnard and Gill 2008). Now consider your assumptions based on the possible reasons for the above statement to see if they fit.

Reasons for 'School shock: parents keep child out of school for six weeks....'	Does this fit with your assumptions?
Child has measles.	
Parents refusing to send a child to school due to bullying.	
School in Britain closed temporarily due to weather damage.	
Child suffering from depression.	

You may see from this exercise that your assumptions on the case were based on your experiences and these did not necessarily fit. Thus, demonstrating how your own interpretations may not always be correct. They are influenced by your own frame of reference, your knowledge and cultural experiences. Likewise the person you are communicating with is also influenced by these. The role that one assumes within the communication is important. In this above scenario the role of the nurse renders them responsible for communicating a healthcare message, whereas a person assuming a patient role becomes dependent in the situation.

Understanding influencing factors in the communication process

In order to more fully understand the communication process, and possible barriers to it, it becomes clear then that a more detailed understanding, rather than the simple model of message/sender/receiver is required. The circular understanding of communication (Arnold and Underman Boggs 2011) discussed in Chapter 1 portrays communication more holistically and takes account of influencing factors both within people and the environment. It outlines how a context also influences the communication process specifically:

- distracting stimuli,
- the communication channels chosen, and
- interpersonal space.

All of the above factors can influence the message being imparted, and/or the sender /receivers perception. In Chapter 1 distracting stimuli were also referred to as 'noise' (DeVito 2009). The particular context in which you will be operating as a student nurse will contain a range of distracting stimuli or noise.

Exercise

Think of a health care situation. What distracting stimuli or noise can you identify that would interfere with the communication of a message? Write two to three lines.

The communication channel used is also a major influencing factor on the potential for the message to become distorted, thus, the channel itself becomes a barrier. Consider the range of communication that a nurse may be involved with in Table 5.1.

> Communicating with multidisciplinary team members
> Charing meetings and contributing to meetings
> Oral and written patient reports at change of staff periods
> Assessing, planning, evaluating and implementing care
> Communicating with families and relatives and providing information
> Recording interventions such as medication delivery
> Recording patient observations and vital signs
> Communicating with patients and providing information
> Breaking bad news
> Making requests
> Providing updates to the multidisciplinary team on patient status
> Communicating vital timely information about changes in patients condition
> Supporting patients and families
> Communicating to manage the care environment
> Communicating appointments
> Written communication of nursing care delivered
> Email communication
> Phone communication

Table 5.1 Examples of nurse communication in the health care setting.

Exercise

From the list in Table 5.1 describe one type of nurse communication channel and how it operates.

> What distracting stimuli or noise can you identify that would interfere with the communication of a message? Write two to three lines.
> How might the communication itself form a barrier to the communication? Write two to three lines

It is clear that a range of physical, psychological, environmental issues affect communication thus the circular notion of communication (as outlined in Figure 1.1) provides a more detailed outline of what happens when we communicate. Both sender and receiver are influenced by a range of factors these are:

- internal frame of reference,
- knowledge,
- culture,
- communication abilities,
- values, and
- role.

You can see the role that a person takes also influences the communication. For you as a nurse, your professional role will influence how you behave. In particular the professional body that regulates the nursing profession in the country in which you work will guide both the skills of communication that you must exhibit and also particular codes of ethics and conduct.

In the United Kingdom for example, historically from the outset of registration nurses have been expected to exhibit proficiency in communication. The most recent guidelines for preregistration nursing requirements in this regard have made the competence requirements in relation to communication more explicit and detailed than in the past (Nursing and Midwifery Council 2010). They state that:

> All nurses must use excellent communication and interpersonal skills. Their communications must always be safe, effective compassionate and respectful. They must communicate effectively using a wide range of strategies and interventions including the effective use of communication technologies. (National Nursing and Midwifery Council (NMC) 2010: 15)

Furthermore they have outlined a range of competencies that a nurse must possess, one of which is communication. Specifically the nurse must display core competencies within the domain of *communication and interpersonal skills* (NMC 2010). They describe an overarching field competence:

> Adult nurses must demonstrate the ability to listen with empathy. They must be able to respond warmly and positively to people of all ages who may be anxious, distressed, or facing problems with their health and wellbeing. (NMC 2010: 15).

Following on from the broad competence they describe a range of field competencies that nurses are expected to demonstrate within the domain of communication and interpersonal skills such as those outlined in Table 5.2.

Specific communication barriers can exist within the nurse and patient that affect therapeutic communication. Nurse and patient come to the healthcare situation with their own goals and requirements. Communication facilitates a relationship where these goals merge to form mutual goals (Arnold and Underman Boggs 2011). Barriers that exist affect the ability for mutually agreed goals to exist.

Thoughtful, insightful and deliberate focus on the therapeutic relationship by nurses serves to enrich the hospital experience for patients (McCabe 2004). In a cost and quality driven era, the essential and fundamental tasks that relate to the management of each patient may form the priority of care. However, the extension of the nurses' role beyond these tasks, serves to address patients' needs in a more meaningful way.

Specific communication skills outlined in Chapter 4 including non-verbal communication skills (listening and touch) and verbal skills (questioning, information giving and paralinguistics), developing rapport and empathy are essential building blocks of the therapeutic relationship. However, there are many barriers that exist to the effective use of these skills in the practice setting. Furthermore it is often the case that patients don't communicate their needs directly, rather they send subtle messages 'cues' through non-verbal means (Uitterhoeve et al. 2008) and the presence of barriers can make it more difficult to notice these subtleties.

Field competencies

1. All nurses must build partnerships and therapeutic relationships through safe, effective and non-discriminatory communication. They must take account of individual differences, capabilities and needs.

2. All nurses must use a range of communication skills and technologies to support person-centred care and enhance quality and safety. They must ensure people receive all the information they need in a language and manner that allows them to make informed choices and share decision making. They must recognise when language interpretation or other communication support is needed and know how to obtain it.

3. All nurses must use the full range of communication methods, including verbal,non-verbal and written, to acquire, interpret and record their knowledge and understanding of people's needs. They must be aware of their own values and, beliefs and the impact this may have on their communication with others. They must take account of the many different ways in which people communicate and how these may be influenced by ill health, disability and other factors, and be able to recognise and respond effectively when a person finds it hard to communicate.

3.1 *Adult nurses must promote the concept, knowledge and practice of selfcare with people with acute and long-term conditions, using a range of communication skills and strategies.*

4. All nurses must recognise when people are anxious or in distress and respond effectively, using therapeutic principles, to promote their wellbeing, manage personal safety and resolve conflict. They must use effective communication strategies and negotiation techniques to achieve best outcomes, respecting the dignity and human rights of all concerned. They must know when to consult a third party and how to make referrals for advocacy, mediation or arbitration.

5. All nurses must use therapeutic principles to engage, maintain and, where appropriate, disengage from professional caring relationships, and must always respect professional boundaries.

6. All nurses must take every opportunity to encourage health-promoting behaviour through education, role modelling and effective communication.

7. All nurses must maintain accurate, clear and complete records, including the use of electronic formats, using appropriate and plain language.

8. All nurses must respect individual rights to confidentiality and keep information secure and confidential in accordance with the law and relevant ethical and regulatory frameworks, taking account of local protocols. They must also actively share personal information with others

Table 5.2 Field competencies related to the domain of *communication and interpersonal skills* for adult nurses

Source: NMC 2010:15. Reproduced with kind permission from Nursing and Midwifery Council.

As highlighted in Chapter 3, Peplau's (1952, 1991) work resolutely emphasized the interpersonal nature of nursing as contributing to the distinctive role that nursing can offer to healthcare (Aggleton and Chalmers 2000). Peplau (1952, 1991) introduced the idea of the therapeutic relationship as being a human connection that heals. Similarly, the influence of theory principles from other disciplines all serve to influence the proposal of nursing care that should be patient centred (Arnold and Underman Boggs 2011). It is only through good communication skills (see Chapter 4) and the development of the therapeutic relationship (Chapter 3) that nurses truly can identify and respond to the unique needs of their patients in a patient-centred way.

Communication is valued as a fundamental nursing role. Good communication is at the core of the therapeutic relationship that nurses strive to attain with patients in their care. Inadequate use of communication skills presents a barrier to the development of a therapeutic relationship (Keating et al. 2002). Costa (2001) recommended that nurses develop specific *therapeutic* communication skills in order to address patients' needs more fully. This included, being 'truly present' to the patient, manifested by being able to listen, being perceptive to the environment and being able to anticipate the patient's needs. Communication skills deemed fundamental to the therapeutic relationship are: being able to identify individual informational needs, empowering patients and being present to patients (Costa 2001). However barriers exist to the operation of these skills in practice. These can occur within the nurse, within the patient and within the environment. The main barriers that emerge from the literature are now explored.

Barriers in the nurse

Keating et al. (2002) examined barriers to nurse–patient relationships and suggested a need for an improvement in communication skills as they identified poor communication as the principal barrier to the development of the relationship. Within communication skills they reported that the listening skills of nurses in the study featured as the most prominent barrier to communication and relationship development.

When you are listening you really have to show that you are paying attention to others (Hargie 2011). The reasons for this are:

- to convey interest and concern;
- to encourage full, open, honest discussion;
- to show and develop a patient-centred approach; and
- to reach shared agreement.

Nurses do not always display the level of interest required for this empathetic listening, and therefore do not appear to communicate well with patients. This can be due to inattentiveness, individual bias or thinking about what they are going to say next (Hargie 2011). Within all individuals barriers exist to listening such as a preoccupation with what one wishes to say next, or self-consciousness (Sidell 2000). This latter element is a preoccupation with oneself during the communication, thus, for example, precipitating thoughts about the next job to be done. This can deflect from the focus on the individual who is actually talking. Other recognized barriers include stress, anxiety, poor attention, misinterpretations and the use of 'rehearsing responses' (Burnard 1997).

As indicated in Chapter 4, good listening skills are essential requisites of nursing. Sometimes the nurse is not just listening to what is being said, but how it is conveyed so that subtle emotional reactions can be interpreted (Uitterhoeve et al. 2008). Poor listening skills were also uncovered by Costa (2001). Uitterhoeve et al. (2008) found that nurses were often unable to respond adequately to patients' emotional expressions: most distanced themselves from patients as a response and few demonstrated empathy. In Costa's (2001) study a nurse casually dismissed a patient who expressed a fear of dying during surgery. Clearly, the item was heard but the patient's real feelings, fears and needs in this particular area were not attended to. Albeit one situation, this clearly highlights the major omissions that can occur if active listening is not carried out. Patients want to be listened to and to be involved in their care. Coyle and Williams (2001: 456) recommended 'asking patients regularly about their feelings and views and encouraging them to ask questions ... to clarify the extent to which they what to be involved [in their care]'.

Using listening skills in conjunction with questioning skills and observing patient cues allows the nurse to operate truly patient-centred communication. While generalized barriers to effective listening are common, nurses and other healthcare settings have a unique responsibility to listen to patients to ascertain patient reactions, questions needs and problems. It is essential that nurses use *active* listening and make a deliberate and conscious effort to listen to the patient, hear and recognize what is being said and plan care accordingly.

Active listening is not an automatic passive behaviour. True active listening involves more than just hearing (Burnard 1997). It involves a range of behaviours, such as using prompts or phrases to encourage the other person to speak more and observation of a variety of non-verbal cues. It involves reflection on what is being said and understanding the person's perspective (Arnold and Underman Boggs 2011). Sidell (2000) noted that: a failure to align oneself opposite and proximal to the patient (sitting or standing); a failure to provide an appropriate venue or time; the absence of interested facial expression or nodding of the head; and a lack of open posture may all demonstrate that the nurse is not paying attention to what the patient has to say. There is failure to attend. These processes are covered in more detail in Chapter 4.

Barriers to active listening may result from a failure to fully engage with the patient. While the nurse may appear to be listening, the absence of adjunct non-verbal behaviours that support active listening including the use of appropriate body postures and gestures by the nurse may give conflicting messages. For example, in McCabe's (2004) study the nurses gave an impression of being busy through non-verbal means and a 'lack of communication' was an emerging theme. It was communicated clearly (although not verbally) to all of these patients that the nurse was too busy to talk. The participants in this study frequently said that nurses did not provide enough information and many commented on how nurses were more concerned with tasks rather than with talking with them. However, all the participants felt that it was not the nurse's fault as they were too "busy'.

It is important, in a busy rushed environment, to give time, or at least the perception of time for the patient. Rather than appearing busy or action orientated the use of attending skills when listening increases the likelihood of reducing barriers that exist. Attending behaviour was described as the physical demonstration of nurses' accessibility and readiness to listen to patients through the use of non-verbal communication.

Attending is a skill that is valued highly by patients. Indeed it was an emerging theme in McCabe's (2004) study. Although the participants of this study did not refer directly to the term 'attending', they described nursing behaviours they valued that were specific to attending. These behaviours were elucidated as 'giving time and being there', 'open/honest communication' and 'genuineness'. 'Being there' was also an emergent theme in O'Brien's (2000) study. In addition to its function within attending the *presence* of the nurses in studies (O'Brien 2000; Costa 2001; McCabe 2004) involved self-disclosure, genuineness and empathy. This empathetic understanding, as Corbett (2001) described it, is a special dimension in the building of a caring relationship that fundamentally comprises of acceptance and respect without prejudice and also without any inference of agreement or disagreement, approval or disapproval, simply to perceive the world as the patient does.

Coyle and Williams (2001) study of 97 patients from general wards found that patients required:

- more involvement in care,
- more information,
- increased sensitivity by staff to the impact of their illness and treatment on their life, and
- an increased approachability of staff.

Sometimes it seems that nurses only approach patients to deal with administrative or functional activities, thus a high level of interest in speaking with patients is not necessarily displayed. Students too, while they are learning, have been found to have display communication skills that are quite task focused. According to Suikkala et al. (2009) facilitative communication focuses on the common good of both the student and the patient (for further details see Chapter 3 this volume) and clearly a facilitative approach is desired although Gibbons (1993) suggested that nurses find this difficult as their work is so action oriented. However, in the United Kingdom one palliative care team (Wilkinson et al. 2008b) expressed dedication to improving nurse patient communication by providing further education and training. The effect of this improved nurses' confidence and an improvement in communication with patients was also noted. A similar approach with cardiac nurses also improved nurses' skills (Wilkinson et al. 2008a).

Professional requirements suggest that nurses should be able to communicate effectively with patients and recognize and alleviate barriers to effective communication (An Bord Altranais 2010: 6), thus training courses to address skill deficits are important (Wilkinson et al. 2008a, 2008b; Fallowfield et al. 2002). However, nurses may undervalue communication in the healthcare setting and may be unaware of the meaning and significance of the nurse–patient relationship for patients (Jarrett and Payne 2000). This lack of awareness may result in nurses making assumptions about what nursing care a patient needs or wants because they do often not ask patients (McCabe 2004). Additionally patients often do not directly state their needs and rely on the nurses' skilled communication to interpret complex emotions, particularly in end of life care (Wilkinson et al. 2008b). The result of ineffective communication and lack of awareness of its importance can be blocking by nurses or superficial communication (Wilkinson et al. 2008a). Active listening is essential in patient-centred communication although the barriers to listening that exist in the healthcare context can be addressed through education and training (Wilkinson et al. 2008a, 2008b; Fallowfield et al. 2002).

Interestingly although there is little research on this topic, the look of the nurse may also influence the nurse/patient encounter. Patients expect a nurse to be professional. Appropriate dress and appearance are thought to portray and communicate an air of professionalism to patients and foster trust. Kalb et al. (2006: 138) noted that:

dress is expected to be neat, respectful, professional, modest, comfortable and designed to allow the nurse to perform the required job duties. Some examples of inappropriate dress include worn, ripped, frayed, torn or unkempt clothing. Also, items that display obscene, profane, discriminatory, provocative or inflammatory words/pictures are not acceptable.

In Kalb et al.'s (2006) view messages displayed on clothing can inadvertently send the wrong message to patients, and as representatives of the health organization nurses are not permitted to wear offensive clothing. Thus responsibility has been taken to ensure that barriers to nurse–patient communication are not amplified by inappropriate dress. DeVito (2011: 103) suggests that 'clothing and body adornment' sends messages to others, which he terms 'artefactual communication'. Unkempt hair, for example, may communicate a 'lack of interest in appearances' and body piercing can convey an unwillingness to conform (DeVito 2011: 103). Both can reduce people's perception of a person's credibility (DeVito 2011). While there has been a lot of change and modernization in nursing uniform in recent decades, to comply with comfort and safety requirements, regulations about neatness and cleanliness of nurses' appearance should not be deemed an historical tradition or ritual that can be abandoned in light of modernization. A nurses' appearance communicates a lot to the public, and this needs to be considered to ensure that you dress suitably for the roles that you undertake.

Barriers exist within the nurse first due to a natural reliance on a personal frame of reference. Additionally failure to listen and a concern with task may serve as barriers to good communication and forming therapeutic relationships with patients. To overcome this you need to become aware of the possibility of barriers forming within the context of communication, and also the key elements of good communication:

- appropriate self-disclosure,
- genuineness,
- empathy,
- emphatic listening,
- being present, and
- professional attire.

Attitudes, values and beliefs

The nurse's attitudes, values and beliefs influence communication (Hindle 2006). The beliefs of the nurse in Edwards (1998) study (who considered the patient's touch to be sexual) directly affected her behaviour towards that patient (anger). Similarly, touch practices in general appeared to be strongly influenced by attitudes, values and beliefs originating within the nurse's own family of origin. Prejudices were another psychological factor identified by Hindle (2006) that can affect nurse–patient communication. Prejudice involves 'making assumptions about people and attributing certain labels and stereotypes to them' (Hindle, 2006: 53).

Kirkham et al. (2002) described the use of stereotyping as a defence mechanism used by midwives to cope with their professional role. They found that midwives sometimes misjudged women's ability and willingness to participate in their maternity care and, as a consequence, women were negatively labelled, for example, as demanding and/or as uncooperative. Midwives often formulated their opinions about their clients on the basis of circumstances over which childbearing women exercised little control: housing tenure, age and/or social class. Even when such judgments were shown to be erroneous, they generally endured throughout the maternity episode. They suggest that stereotyping by nurses, although possibly a way of coping in a situation with limited resources, was 'corrosive' in that it affected the therapeutic relationship, particularly in relation to choice and decision making.

Similarly, Somali women in Davies and Bath's (2001) study perceived that they were denied information due to punitive attitudes and prejudiced views among health professionals. Likewise, Bowler (1993) investigated the delivery of maternity care to women of South Asian descent in Britain using an ethnographic approach. She found that the midwives commonly held stereotypical views of women. Their stereotype of women of Asian descent contained four main themes: communication problems; failure to comply with care and service abuse; making a fuss about nothing; and a lack of normal maternal instinct.

Prejudice commonly, although not exclusively, occurs in ethnic minority groups. The older person may also encounter this (Williams et al. 2004) whereby assumptions are made about hospitalized older people (that they are cognitively impaired and require 'baby talk' as a form of communication). Similarly those with mental illness may also experience prejudice. A study conducted in Durban, South Africa, found that 90 per cent of the nurses in a general hospital setting held negative attitudes toward people with mental illnesses (Mavundla and Uys, 1997). Jorm et al. (1999) reported that health professionals were more likely than the general public to discriminate against those with mental illness. Similarly, Foster and Onyeukwu (2003) reported negative attitudes in forensic nurses towards substance misuse in the mentally ill. Prejudice can also exist towards those whose sexual orientation differs from that of the nurse, although attitudes towards lesbians and gay men do appear to be more positive than previously reported (Röndahl et al. 2004). Similarly, those experiencing certain illness such as HIV/AIDS can experience prejudice (Cree et al. 2004).

As a profession working in a multicultural society nurses and midwives ought to be able to respond to these needs appropriately. Great care must be taken to explore and reflect upon personal attitudes and behaviour when nursing all patients. Through self-awareness and personal development (Chapter 9) these issues can be addressed. This is important because these can form significant barriers to communication in a healthcare context and to the overall aim of developing a therapeutic relationship with patients. Developing an empathetic understanding of individuals may help to overcome this. Listening skills can also be improved through self-awareness and personal development. Seeking educational opportunities is also important.

The nurse is but one aspect of the nurse–patient relationship and barriers also exist within patients.

Barriers within patients

Those patients who do not speak the native language of a country face additional barriers to engaging effectively in communication. Poor communication between non-English speaking Somali women and health workers was identified as a problem in Davies and Bath's (2001) study and restricted women's information seeking behaviour. Even though interpreters were provided, fears about misinterpretation and confidentiality restricted the women's use of this service.

The presence and use of written instructions and information leaflets in a variety of relevant languages can be useful in overcoming the language barrier. However, it is important that these are developed with the patient in mind and avoid overuse of sophisticated language. The patient's ethnic origin and previous experience of reading are also crucial. Illiteracy is an identified barrier to learning and with much communication relying upon written materials it can cause problems for the patient (Doak et al. 1985). Even where there is no illiteracy as such, many educational reading materials are written at a level that presents reading difficultly to the average patient (Zion and Aiman 1989). An accurate assessment of the patient's reading ability is required to ensure that these learning tools are useful. However, this is not always possible, as patients may not admit to a reading difficulty. It is important therefore that nursing staff reinforce written information with verbal information and involve members of the family.

Unequal power relationships

Earlier in the chapter we discussed the variety of responses that patients may have to the use of touch and cautioned against routine use without first establishing a patient's view and need within the context of the therapeutic relationship. This area reveals patient vulnerability with regard to communication. This may be attributed to the depersonalization and subordination of patients as individuals while in care. Edward's (1998) notion of the subordinate patient in the nurse/patient touch scenario needs to be borne in mind. In many clinical situations the power base often rests with the health care workers and not the patient.

These issues identify potentially important barriers to effective communication in the healthcare setting. Morrall (2003) described the social factors affecting communication under the headings freedom, power, sickness and social discourse. The relationship with a patient who is a recipient of healthcare is socially constructed and the patient may be in a dependent role. As demonstrated in many of the studies, patients may receive a pat on the head, whether they like it or not demonstrating the effect of the social construction of healthcare in some settings where patients are not equal partners in decisions affecting their care. Likewise the potential power exerted by nurses is evidenced in its use for persuasion purposes (Edwards 1998). Furthermore adopting the 'sick role' that Morrall (2003) described may contribute to the patient's acceptance of touch as part of their healthcare experience.

The construction of unequal power relationships, the social construction of health and illness and the potential adoption of the 'sick role' can all affect communication in the healthcare setting (Morrall 2003).

The likely affect of these factors is that the patient may not be able to engage fully in a therapeutic relationship due to their perceived dependence and lack of autonomy. They may not act as equal partners in their care and become passive recipients of care.

Overcoming barriers

It is essential that nurses explore current methods of communication delivery, existent barriers and methods for overcoming these, particularly in the presence of additional barriers such as language and hearing loss. Communication and the therapeutic nurse–patient relationship situation is not an esoteric element of nursing, but rather a fundamental aspect of caring. It is within this context that improvements in this area need to be considered. Areas that may be considered include family involvement, nursing theory and conceptual model use. Developing self-awareness and using reflection are other tools to identify and deal with barriers to communication and these are explored in Chapters 9 and 10.

Family involvement

The therapeutic relationship, partnership and empowerment are not confined to the patient. The client does not live in the world in isolation, but rather as a part of a family, community and environment. It is increasingly being recognized that the social support has an important role in the dynamic between patient and nurse, and in the past this vital aspect of patient care has often been overlooked. The diversity of the patient's social support requires acceptance and identification in the healthcare context. Social support from others outside the healthcare setting is a perceived source of comfort for patients. A sense of comfort was noted from previous studies of day surgery by the presence of family members both preoperatively and post-operatively, and showed a significant effect on the patients' perceived sense of social support (Wheeler 2010). Driscoll (2000) also found that the inclusion of carers when information is given to the patients improved the level of satisfaction with information given thus reducing the carer's anxiety after discharge and also decreased the possibility of experiencing any medical problems at home. Simons and Robertson (2002) found that parents were in a good position to act as advocates for their children. The obvious benefits from family involvement need to be incorporated into practice. Allowing the attendance of some family members where possible may a source of comfort and facilities for this should be provided. At a more fundamental level, the vital communication skills that are fundamental to the therapeutic relationship need to be extended to the family to provide a holistic approach to care. Wheeler (2010) found that nurses caring for older people with dementia found that 'involving family and the keeping family on board' was crucial to good communication with patients.

Education

There is no substitute, however, for education and training, which is known to improve communication skills. Indeed, Chambers-Evans et al. (1999) found that the experience gained by nurses participating in a qualitative research interview training project helped nurses to obtain a deeper understanding of nurse–patient communication by utilizing skills such as listening, understanding and validating responses. It is imperative therefore that nurses and employers explore communication training options available to them. Betts (2001) identified education as crucial to improving nurses' communication skills and highlighted a deficit in skills training.

Keating et al. (2002), who identified barriers to nurse–patient relationships among 119 nurses in Australia, found that communication was identified as the principal barrier to the development of the relationship.

Education can have a positive effect on the communication skills of nurses (Chambers-Evans et al. 1999). However, the lack of good communication suggests the need for a holistic framework to guide and direct nursing practice in this area (Betts 2001). From a systematic review of the literature Michie et al. (2003) identified the ability to elicit and discuss patients' beliefs and the ability to activate the patient to take control as integral components of such a model. Similarly, Fossum and Arborelius (2004) identified that, in an observation study of outpatient doctor/patient interactions, involving the patient in management led to more successful communication. Fossum and Arborelisu (2004) also amalgamated the findings of previous studies into suggestions to improve patient-centred communication. These recommendations included:

- Providing the opportunity for the patient to express their needs, including symptoms, thoughts, feelings and expectations.
- Treating the patient as a person with a health need, rather than the perception of the person as a disease entity.
- Ensuring that the patient feels that they have been understood.

Gallant et al. (2002) reiterated that clients often develop sophisticated knowledge about how to manage their illness. It has been found that consumers of healthcare value the process of shared decision making whereby they feel respected and make a meaningful contribution to the discussions as well as clear arrangements for a review of the treatment decisions (Edwards et al. 2003).

It is from this perspective that the concept of partnership can be introduced into the modern healthcare system as a way of overcoming barriers to communication. The therapeutic relationship fulfils the criteria of a partnership as it reflects an interpersonal relationship between two or more people towards mutually defined goals (Gallant et al. 2002). The roles and responsibilities of the partners may vary during this partnership. In essence the nurse promotes client empowerment and competency by sustaining the relationship and reinforcing client progress, supporting decision -making and assisting the client to develop more knowledge and skills (Gallant et al. 2002).

Nursing theory and conceptual model use

Nursing theory and conceptual model use, as described in Chapter 2, also provides a way forward for overcoming barriers to communication in the practice setting. Partnership in the nurse–patient relationship with recognition of patient autonomy is a recurring theme throughout popular nursing theory (Pearson et al. 2005). The development of a nurse/patient relationship was a fundamental component of Peplau's (1952, 1991) work. This particular aspect of nursing has particular relevance for moving away from the medical, traditional and routine models of care (Pearson et al. 2005).

A lack of individualization of care is a barrier to communication. Conceptual models have contributed much to the individualization of nursing (Tierney 1998). Roper et al. (2001) emphasized the individual nature of this process of nursing and the necessity for patient participation, all elements of what we may begin to consider as patient-centred care. Their model also allows for specific assessment of individual needs and problems in activities of living (ALs) and may be said to facilitate patient-centred communication.

Partnership is an explicit aspect of the use of the Self-Care Nursing theory (SCNT) as a conceptual model in practice (Orem 2001). Empowerment is also crucial. Rather than nursing care being regarded solely as providing direct care to another, Orem (2001) also highlighted the important nursing actions of supporting and educating patients. The development of the nurse–patient relationship was identified as crucial to this process (Orem 2001) as essential for the full and participative involvement of patients in care.

The identified barriers that exist may be also be related to an underpinning lack of communication skills. One of the fundamental values that should underpin today's nursing practice is the development of a therapeutic relationship between nurse and patient (Arnold and Underman Boggs 2011). This relationship is emphasized throughout the literature on the topic (Aggleton and Chalmers 2000). It is only through good communication and the development of the therapeutic relationship that nurses can truly identify the unique needs of their patients and address potential barriers. This process underpins contemporary approaches to communication within healthcare settings (Ito and Lambert 2002) and supports a nurse–patient communication that is patient centred.

In today's accelerated healthcare environment, where cost and quality issues predominate, we must not lose sight of the fundamental communication skills required by nurses. At the heart of nursing is caring. Recent studies indicate the high value that patients place on the presence of the nurse. It is essential that nurses value their own unique contribution to the healthcare setting and through personal awareness reflect and build on their communication skills. It is only through the provision of a relationship where the nurse listens to patients and addresses their unique needs that true quality care can be achieved.

Key points

▶ Many barriers exist to the effective development and use of core communication skills in nursing. These barriers can be within the nurse, within the patient or within the environment.

▶ Barriers within the nurse include: a lack of communication skills, undervaluing communication as an integral part of nursing and a lack of awareness of the meaning and significance of nurse–patient communication in providing high quality patient-centred care.

▶ A nurse's personal values, beliefs, attitudes and prejudices can adversely affect the nurse–patient relationship.

▶ Patient-centredness and shared decision making are regarded as key factors in preventing barriers to effective and positive communication.

6 Conflict

Introduction

In this chapter we introduce to you the concept of assertive behaviour. This is an important skill in nursing as it enables you to understand how to interact with patients and staff in a way that does not offend the other person. This is crucial for developing therapeutic relationships as discussed in Chapter 5 but also for developing and maintaining good relationships within a multidisciplinary team. Assertive behaviour is about standing up for your rights (Hargie 2011) and although this may seem a strong statement for a caring profession it is increasingly recognized that being assertive in nursing practice makes a positive contribution to good communication and relationships (Hargie 2011). These skills are also considered integral to allowing nurses to communicate within a multidisciplinary team as an advocate for patients and working collaboratively in a multidisciplinary team.

The nature of interpersonal conflict

Conflict can occur within an individual (intrapersonal), between individuals (interpersonal) within a group (intragroup) or between groups (intergroup) (Balzer-Riley, 2011). Interpersonal conflict occurs when there is a disagreement between or among individuals and arises due to a difference in desired goals or outcomes (Arnold and Underman Boggs 2011). Arnold and Underman Boggs (2011: 272–3) describe interpersonal conflict as 'Tension arising from incompatible goals or needs, in which the actions of one frustrate the ability of the other to achieve their goals, resulting in stress or tension'.

Arnold and Underman Boggs identified common causes of interpersonal conflict as:

- misunderstanding,
- poor communication skills,
- stress,
- personality clashes, and
- value or goal differences.

Conflict situations can occur as a result of:

- having your position discounted,
- being requested to provide more information than you are
- comfortable with,
- being pressured to give more than you can,
- encountering harassment,
- being personally targeted,
- wanting to continue doing things the same way (Arnold and Underman Boggs 2011),
- speaking in an accusing or blaming manner,
- offering unmeant sympathy or false reassurance,
- demonstrating a lack of understanding of a patient/clients perspective,
- exerting pressure to affect a behaviour change, or
- being authoritarian (Arnold and Underman Boggs 2011).

✎ Exercise

Consider the conflict that might occur in a house that you are sharing with two friends. As a nursing student you may have exams over a particular period or may be working long hours and may wish the house to be very quiet. Your personal goal is to achieve your personal study and have sufficient rest to enable to you work effectively for the remainder of your shifts. However your flatmates have finished all their exams and don't attend clinical practice as part of their university course. Their goals vary. Mark wishes to take a break and enjoy himself after months of difficult course work. He feels this is a well-deserved break and is playing noisy computer games and music in his room and is very reluctant to stop when you ask. Lauren

> enjoys reading and is usually fairly quiet but has a flute exam coming up and needs to practice. When you ask her about keeping it down, while she understands your predicament she explains that she must practice.
>
> Think about this situation and write down the type of reaction you might have. Write two to three lines.

This exercise demonstrates how easily conflict can occur when people's personal goals are at variance with one another. It also shows that conflict is an inevitable part of life and a natural occurrence in human relationships (Arnold and Underman Boggs 2011). However, conflict can have either negative or positive outcomes (DeVito 2011). If in the exercise above you decided to keep quiet about your needs so as not to affect the others too much, well then you might end up feeling hurt because your own needs were not met, and others did not seem to understand them. Other negative consequences of conflict include becoming shut off from others, resentment and arguing (DeVito 2011). On the other hand conflict can have positive effects (DeVito 2011). It can build up your confidence in dealing with issues and your relationships may be stronger for having faced up to the conflict. Balzer-Riley (2011: 324) concurs that conflict is a natural part of human interactions and suggests that 'it can be a positive force in nursing if used for growth'.

Interpersonal conflict typically occurs in situations where:

- Individuals are interdependent and connected in some significant way so that the actions of one affect the other (consider the house sharing situation above: each individual's actions affect the others through the connection of living together).
- People are aware that their goals differ or oppose the other person's/people's goals and appear 'mutually incompatible' (it's either one or the other). (In the situation described above the silence required was not compatible with the need for Mark to unwind and for Lauren to prepare for her music exam).

- People feel that the other's goals are interfering with theirs (DeVito 2011:160) (the above scenario displays how each flatmate's goal can interfere with the others' goal).

Think back to your reaction to the exercise above, what did you do? If you became angry or upset with your flatmates, then an argument may have occurred and your flatmates feelings might get have got hurt. If you did nothing both your work and study may have been affected and you could begin to feel demoralized. In general where conflict is not handled well, demoralization and decreased motivation can occur. If you suggested that you might talk things through and try to reach a compromise, then this was a good answer that would hopefully prevent conflict because while differences in goals is a common occurrence it does not always have to result in interpersonal conflict. Very often it is poor communication that results in conflict (Brinkett 2010).

As with all interpersonal relationships interpersonal conflict occurs in nursing and is an inherent feature of complex human systems such as healthcare and is thought to be neither good nor bad (Brinkett 2010). It can occur: within and among nurses; among nurses and other health care professionals; and among nurses, patients and patient's families (Brinkett 2010). Where there is interdependency, as clearly occurs between staff, and between patients and nurses, conflict is bound to occur (Balzer-Riley 2011). However conflict in nursing occurs most commonly between nurses and between nurses and other healthcare professionals, and is reported less frequently with patients (Brinkett 2010). Physician nurse conflict commonly occurs within ethical decision situations such as those that occur during end of life care and also in the operating theatre department (Brinkett 2010). Conflicts can occur about facts, methods, goals and values. Conflict also arises due to differences in professional opinion or through changes in roles: 'As the role of the staff nurse changes, especially during organisational restructuring, role ambiguity may result from unclear job descriptions' (Milstead 1996: 39)

Inadequate communication in terms of a lack of information provided can be a cause of conflict (Milstead 1996). This can result in intrapersonal conflict (conflict within oneself) and interpersonal conflict (conflict with other members of the healthcare team) (Milstead 1996). Nurses are working in an ever-changing environment. As change occurs and roles change, receiving clear up-to-date information about changes, expectations and happenings is crucial in preventing conflict (Milstead 1996). However, Brinkett (2010) highlighted that conflict in the healthcare context can be costly in terms of quality care outcomes, and can result in errors and poor quality care. The exercise above may have given you some idea of how you might personally respond to conflict and it is useful to understand some terminology around conflict responses so that you may begin to develop and improve your own responses and identify responses in others.

Common responses to conflict

Five styles commonly used in response to conflict are avoidance, competition, accommodation and collaboration (Arnold and Underman Boggs 2011).

Exercise

Think about your responses to the exercise above and consider which of the following four styles your response fits into:

1. avoidance,
2. compete,
3. accommodate, or
4. collaborate.

Write two to three lines.

Avoidance involves ignoring the situation and not addressing the issue. If you avoid the conflict this could mean that you simply ignore the problem, or avoid the people involved. In the exercise above you might decide to stay in your room so that you never have to face your neighbours. While this may seem an extreme reaction, avoidance is the most commonly used response to conflict and nurses certainly use this approach as a resolution method.

Competing is usually characterized by aggressive or unco-operative behaviour. You may decide to play your own favourite music loudly while you are studying, which would be very off-putting for the others who both have their own goals and needs, which loud music would affect. Accommodating may result in a quick closure, as you are inclined to give in (you might reluctantly agree to study at night, or go to sleep at your mother's house while you are on night duty) however, this accommodation means that none of your needs are being met and ultimately resentment can build up. While accommodating behaviour is a cooperative approach, it is not really assertive behaviour and arises from a desire to smooth over conflict (Arnold and Underman Boggs 2011).

These behaviours (avoidance, accommodating and competing) are used regularly in everyday interactions. As a nurse a collaborative approach to conflict resolution is most effective. It involves using problem-solving skills, cooperation and open communication. These are all important social skills not only for the healthcare professional but for all aspects of life.

Collaborating means that both sides enter into an open discussion, everything is 'put on the table' and the solution is reached together. The issue or conflict is addressed directly. It starts by setting out and identifying what the problem is, and opening it up for discussion. Then possible solutions are explored that aim to suit everybody in some way, if that is possible, or if accommodation is needed that this is mutually agreed.

Exercise

Think again about the exercise above where Mark and Lauren's behaviours are affecting your study and sleep requirements.

Write out the steps required for collaboration to occur.

The focus in collaboration is on the mutual solving of problems, rather than defeating the other party. It is a solution-oriented response resulting in a mutually satisfying resolution to the problem (Arnold and Underman Boggs 2011). In the exercise you should have provided some answers that require you to sit down with Mark and Lauren, perhaps arranging to meet over a meal. You might have suggested beginning by outlining your position and how important your studies and sleep are currently. You might then say:

> Lauren and Mark I know how important music is to both of you, but I wondered whether we might talk about ways that we could work together to see if there is some way of working in the house that suits everyone.

It is very important when having such discussions to remain unemotional and to stick to the point. This means that even though you may be feeling anxious about your exams, or angry that your friends are not accommodating you and perhaps disturbing you, you still ought not to demonstrate your emotions during the discussion. Showing anger may affect your attempts at collaboration. From your open discussion you might arrive at the following solutions:

- A timetable for noisy music/practice and scheduled quiet times.
- Lauren and Mark are away for two weekends that you were unaware of, and this frees up some quiet study time for you.
- In agreement that Lauren and Mark will practice/play music for four evenings a week you agree to study early in the day for the other three.

Collaboration promotes effective communication and problem solving because both individuals try to seek mutual agreeable solutions. It is amazing the number of interesting solutions that arise simply from sitting down and talking. When collaborating, both parties set aside their original goals and work together to establish a supraordinate or common goal. Despite working on collaborative solutions sometime conflict does arise and you need to be able to deal effectively with it.

Dealing with conflict

Nurses often are required deal with conflict in the work place (Milstead 1996). Resolving conflict requires you to:

- Identify the conflict issues.
- Be aware of your own response to conflict and manage it.
- Separate the problem from the people involved.
- Stay focused on the issue and on the underlying motivations behind the position the other person takes.
- Identify available options.
- Be aware of established procedures for dealing with issues. (Arnold and Underman Boggs 2011).

While all these seems very straightforward it is actually often quite difficult to work out exactly what is going on and what the issues are (Arnold and Underman Boggs 2011). Furthermore our own emotions and perhaps past experiences with the people involved may cloud the issue. What is helpful is to take a piece of paper, and using the stages above to try to identify the specific issues that are at stake. Remember to be honest about your own feelings and identifying these on paper may help you to remain more objective when dealing with the issue. Separating the person from the issue often proves quite difficult. If we take the example from the exercise above that we have been dealing with and add the information that Mark has been playing loud music persistently since you moved in together (two-and-a-half years ago) and persistently forgets his keys so you end up having to let him in at least twice a week. During your attempts at collaboration you will have to (despite the history) keep the discussion focused on the issue at hand, which is getting quiet time for study/sleep during an eight-week period until the summer. Bringing up all the other elements of Mark's behaviour that bother you (even though they are true) is likely to elicit a negative response from Mark. The issue is not about 'Mark' it is about your need for quiet, so avoid personalizing the issue.

Conflict resolution requires:

- consideration of contributory factors,
- consideration of problem solving techniques, and
- active listening.

Even though you are quite keen to have your way (and get a quiet house) you do really need to do some thinking in order for a collaborative solution to work. Think about Mark and Lauren and why they behave in the way they do and try to see the world from their point of view. Revise your conversation and possible solutions to solve the problem. When you are talking with them try to listen attentively, even though it may be tempting to keep interrupting with statements like 'but I have exams coming up'. However, using the 'I' in this type of discussion is strongly recommended (DeVito 2011). When you are wording your open discussion it is better to keep the discussion focused on 'I' rather than 'you', for example: '*I* would really like a quiet couple of weeks in the house, how do you guys think I could go about achieving this?', is much better than: '*You* two are always making noise, is there any way you could stop for a couple of weeks?'

It is also important to identify available options for yourself, be aware of established procedures for dealing with issues. In the exercise above it might be useful to become aware of the legal aspects of making noise early in the morning and late at night, or the landlord/apartment block rules. It might well be that your housemates comply with this already and without necessarily accommodating them (as they are free to play their music) you may make a decision to study outside these hours. As your day sleeping (when you are working nights) is effectively outside the normal sleeping pattern (thus legislation does not protect you against noise) it may be unreasonable to expect total quiet, therefore potential options for you are: to use ear plugs, exercise before you sleep, avoid tea/coffee beforehand and employ other sleep friendly strategies.

However, sometimes dealing with conflict effectively requires using the option of direct confrontation by speaking with the individuals involved. This should not be avoided if this is the necessary solution. Remember dealing directly with situations will give you more confidence and if issues are addressed appropriately your life will become more manageable. Getting into the habit of avoiding situations is not good. When deciding to speak with someone, it usually requires several stages in order to enact it effectively, so don't be tempted to rush into a discussion especially when you are feeling angry or hurt about it (Milstead 1996). The first phase should be an information seeking-phase where you need to find out more information about the situation and what exactly is going on (Milstead 1996: 40). Consideration of contributory factors is important here, including your own contribution to the conflict.

This is followed by planning an appropriate time and place and for the discussion to occur, do not try to catch people when they are in a hurry or doing something else, try to arrange a specific time (Milstead 1996). This also allows them to prepare. In the situation above, for example, you could say: 'Hi Mark, listen I have loads of exams coming up and I need to ask you guys for advice on how best to plan for them, can we chat over coffee tomorrow?'

This gives Mark a little time to think about the content of the discussion, and ensures that you do not catch him unawares. When you choose to speak about the issue you need to remember to stick closely to the issue and not raise side issues (such as the person's other behaviours as previously discussed), as a focused is more likely to be successful.

Thompson (2009) gives a good example of managing conflict, which is termed the 'RED' approach. This summarizes and incorporates elements of other approaches. You might remember it easily if you think of 'seeing red' to describe being angry. So when you feel angry about an issue think RED and:

- R – recognize the issue as a potential conflict
- E – evaluate the conflict (decide what's going on, seek information, see it from the others perspective, look at policy related to it)
- D – deal with it

Remember after dealing with a situation you still need to keep an eye on the situation, ongoing evaluation is always necessary to monitor the conflict.

Other important elements when trying to deal with conflict are to:

- prepare for the encounter;
- organise your information;
- manage your own anger or anxiety;
- time the encounter;
- put the situation into perspective (Arnold and Underman Boggs 2011);
- use therapeutic communication skills;
- use clear communication;
- take one issue at a time;
- mutually generate some options for resolution; and
- make a request for change of behaviour (Arnold and Underman Boggs 2011).

When applying this to the nurse–patient relationship Arnold and Underman Boggs (2011) suggest assessing the presence of conflict by using nursing strategies to enhance conflict resolution. Arnold and Underman Boggs (2011: 285) outline several strategies for dealing with interpersonal conflict. These included developing assertive skills, demonstrating respect to others, using 'I' statements (rather than 'you'), making statements that are clear, using appropriate pitch and tone, being able to analyze personal feelings in the situation and focus on the present. They also describe how to deal with encounters in nursing practice with angry patients or relatives. They suggest using communication skills to observe for early non-verbal clues: once identified the feeling could be labelled (for example anger). For example you could say 'You seem angry'.

They also suggest that you may give permission for anger within limits. This may be demonstrated by the statement 'it is perfectly understandable that you are angry in this situation'. This also helps the person to own the anger feelings. Acknowledging the person's feelings is an important first step in the resolution process. Rather than the nurse talking excessively or trying to use words to resolve the situation, using communication skills identified earlier in the book, a serious of open questions and attentive listening may elicit why the person is angry. This may be very productive in diffusing the situation. By then identifying what it is that has triggered the anger the nurse may be able to assist the person to develop a simple plan to deal with the situation. Thus, active listening, a key component of the therapeutic relationship, prevents the escalation of conflict (Arnold and Underman Boggs 2011).

Other therapeutic listening responses can also be useful in this situation, such as using minimal cues and avoiding leading questions. Thus rather than saying 'you are annoyed because your visitors had to leave early' you would elicit more information and be less likely to aggravate the situation by using the statement 'tell me what is happening for you right now'. In a conflict situation with a patient or visitor, it is important to use the self-awareness that you have developed to prevent yourself from jumping in and providing a range of responses to the situation. Once a response has been elicited from the open question, it can be clarified, 'so you're telling me that you are cross because visiting time seemed to be very short today', summarized or paraphrased. Silence can also be used if appropriate. The nurse's response must be calm with use of appropriate vocabulary with a view to focusing the situation on the problem and presenting reality. In this case, the short visiting times may be unavoidable and this could be explained. However, providing empathy in a situation of disappointment might serve to ease the tension. Similarly, there may be room for an apology if the visitor was rushed away in a manner that was not appropriate.

Arnold and Underman Boggs (2011: 193) also suggested using humour, which they describe as 'a powerful communication technique when it is used with deliberate intent for a specific therapeutic purpose'. Humour would obviously need to be used appropriately, but can be used to show one's authentic self and can diffuse tension in some situations.

Rosenblatt and Davis (2009) suggest that nurses should use self-development to improve their conflict resolution skills. They suggest practicing a forthcoming difficult communication by taping oneself with a recording device (Rosenblatt and Davis 2009). This recording may be analyzed to see how it might be improved before the interaction. The focus of any analysis should be to determine whether the interaction was (or will be) person centred or not. When analyzing a situation you should consider the extent to which you exhibited the following behaviours:

- approachability,
- respect to the other person,
- friendliness,
- appropriate humour,
- openness,
- willingness to listen, and
- evidence of having listened and taken the person seriously.

Conflict is regarded as a natural part of the clinical environment within which many nurses and nursing students operate (Balzer-Riley 2011). It can have positive outcomes and be of benefit to situations if it is handled assertively (Balzer-Riley 2011). Resolution of conflict in workplace situation means acting in such a way that agreement is reached that is acceptable and pleasing to all parties. Balzer-Riley (2011) suggests assertiveness as a response to overcome conflict. A nurse who is behaving assertively not only stands up for their own rights, but advocates actively for the rights of others (Balzer-Riley 2011). Using assertive skills will now be explored.

Using assertive skills

Assertiveness is a very important social and communication skill in professional and everyday interactions (Hargie 2011). It is defined as 'setting goals, acting on those goals in a clear, consistent manner and taking responsibility for the consequences of those actions' (Arnold and Underman Boggs (2011: 275). Arnold and Underman Boggs (2011) suggest assertiveness as a suitable way of dealing with conflict. Although commonly thought to be a personality trait, assertiveness is a form of behaviour that can be learned (Hargie 2011). It is also situation specific; thereby its use can be selective (Hargie 2011).

Assertive behaviour:

- is a learned skill and
- involves communicating needs and requests clearly without belittling either person in the communication.

Hargie (2011) suggests that a plethora of research in the area of assertive behaviour has taken place over the past 50 years. They suggested that assertion rose to prominence as a social skill in the mid 1970s as a pop psychology fad and as a clinical focus of behaviour therapy. Assertion and assertive behaviour are also gaining increasing popularity within the nursing literature.

Assertiveness involves specific responses to situations including:

- admitting your own shortcomings (self-disclosure),
- giving and receiving compliments,
- initiating and maintaining interactions,
- expressing positive feelings,
- expressing unpopular or different opinions,
- requesting behaviour changes by others, and
- refusing unreasonable requests.

The goals of assertiveness are (Hargie 2011):

- To protect personal rights.
- To withstand unreasonable requests.
- To make reasonable requests.
- To deal with unreasonable refusals.
- To recognise the personal rights of others.
- To change the behaviour of others.
- To avoid unnecessary conflicts.
- To confidently communicate position.

Why be assertive?

- To stand up for yourself and your rights without infringing others' rights.
- To reduce anxiety as anxiety can prevent assertiveness (Arnold and Underman Boggs 2011).
- Patient advocacy (Timmins and McCabe 2005).

Assertive behaviour involves four components.

1. Being able to say 'no' assertively.
2. Being able to ask for what you want, without compromising the other.

3. Appropriately express positive and negative thoughts and feelings.
4. Initiate, continue and terminate interaction (Arnold and Underman Boggs 2011).

There are also barriers to assertive behaviour that include:

- a lack of practice,
- no formative training and no role models,
- being unclear,
- a fear of hostility,
- undervaluing yourself,
- poor presentation,
- a lack of knowledge about personal and professional rights,
- an anxiety due to a lack of self-esteem and confidence, and
- concern about what others will think.

When we speak about assertive behaviour these are usually considered in the context of four different response styles:

- Aggressive: talking at others, may lead to counter-aggression.
- Assertive: talking with others.
- Manipulative: attempt to subvert with charm and/flattery.
- Submissive: talking little to others.

Responses to conflict

Aggressive responses

Aggressive responses involve an attempt to use personal anger to persuade the other person. This can involve body language such as proximity (standing too close to another) or finger wagging. Taylor (1989) suggested that this should not be confused with anger. Expressing anger can be useful in a situation, and may be done assertively, for example, by saying in a normal voice tone: 'I feel angry that I have to work next Sunday, I had made prior arrangements'. However, in this response the person is simply expressing their feelings openly without expecting the other to act. When aggression is used there is a deliberate attempt to persuade or punish the other individual in the interaction.

The use of a loud voice and aggressive body language (finger wagging, standing over the other) all contribute to the aggressive message. Passive responses on the other hand are aimed at quiet manipulation. This could include withdrawal, for example, refusing to contribute to a team meeting or quietly refusing to implement new ways of working. The defensive response according to Taylor (1989) is where individuals have a sense of belonging over something, territory, equipment or regulations. At the slightest imposition the person rises to defend, without considering the other's viewpoint and it can quickly escalate into aggression. Willis and Daisley (1995) described aggression as seeking to get your own way regardless of the consequences. This can be indirect and not that obvious or loud, violent and abusive with interruptions and intimidation common. The results of aggression are arguments are won at the expense of others, people are annoyed and the person may be disliked and freaked.

The manipulative response

The manipulative response Taylor (1989) suggested is one of the most common responses to conflict, particularly in situations and cultures where open conflict or direct confrontation is discouraged. Those using manipulation try to take the focus away from the person who is trying to express an opinion. By changing the topic, minimizing or scoffing at the suggestion the subject is inevitably changed. This behaviour 'frustrate[s] the efforts of others into giving up on an issue' (Taylor 1989: 26).

The passive response

Passive behaviour Willis and Daisley (1995 p.10) suggested, is keeping quiet so as not to upset others, keeping thoughts and

Assertive behaviour:
- Being open and honest with yourself and other people
- Listening to other people's point of view
- Showing an understanding of other people's situations
- Expressing your ideas clearly, but not at the expense of others
- Being able to reach workable solutions to difficulties
- Making decisions – even if your decision is not to make a decision!
- Being clear about your point and not being sidetracked
- Dealing with conflict
- Speaking up
- Having self-respect and respect for other people
- Being equal with others while restating your uniqueness
- Expressing your feelings honestly but with care
- Standing up for yourself

Results of assertive behaviour:
- Conflicts are resolved openly
- Potential difficult situations are dealt with early
- Confidence increases
- Fear reduces as skills are developed in handling emotional situations
- People become equal with others while retaining their uniqueness
- There is recognition of the effect of behaviour on others
- People retain their dignity

Figure 6.1   Assertive behaviour and results

Source: adapted from Willis, L. and Daisley, J. (1995) *The Assertive Trainer: A Practical Handbook for Trainers and Running Assertiveness Courses*, Maidenhead: McGraw-Hill Book Company Europe.

feelings internalized, 'saying yes when you want to say no' excessive apologizing and appearing indecisive while actually knowing what one wants. The results of passive behaviour are that arguments are lost, the person may feel like a doormat or a victim, the person remains indecisive and may become 'bitter later in life' (Willis and Daisley, 1995: 11). The overriding motto of passive behaviour is 'anything for a quiet life' (Willis and Daisley, 1995: 11). Assertive behaviour on the other hand is quite different (Willis and Daisley 1995) and is displayed in Figure 6.1.

The assertive response

Willis and Daisley (1995: 12) described assertive behaviour as 'a form of behaviour which demonstrates your self-respect and respect for others. This means that assertiveness is concerned with dealing with your own feelings about yourself and other people, as much as with the end result'. The five vital ingredients according to Willis and Daisley (1994) are:

- listen,
- demonstrate that you understand the other person,
- say what you think and feel,
- say specifically what you want to happen, and
- consider the consequences for yourself and others of any joint solutions,

They also focused on using 'assertive words' (Willis and Daisley 1995: 24), suggesting that having an understanding of what assertiveness is does not necessarily mean that assertive behaviour will follow.

Assertive words can be used as follows:

- I understand that you think …
- However, I feel …
- Therefore, I suggest …

Exercise

Bring yourself back to your previous exercises dealing with your request for quietness for your studies. Add these assertive words to your imaginary discussion with Lauren and Mark.

- I understand that you think …
- However, I feel …
- Therefore, I suggest …

What would you say?

It is important to speak in a way that is open, clear, constructive and in a voice that is steady, firm, warm, clear, sincere, neither loud nor soft and audible. A voice that is fast, pompous, loud, strident, sharp, abrupt, shouting, clipped or sarcastic that uses excessive emphasis on words, threatening statements or criticism conveys aggression. Whereas being longwinded, apologetic, self-critical with a soft, hesitant, tentative, slow/quiet or fast and garbled approach can appear passive. Your spoken words are 'your assertive script' (Willis and Daisley 1995: 24) and represent only a tiny proportion of the message conveyed. To be assertive not only involves using assertive language but one must '*sound* assertive and *look* assertive whilst delivering them' (Willis and Daisley 1995: 24, emphasis added). This is an important aspect of learning and practicing assertive behaviour skills because even if you use assertive language, if you look and behave angrily then you will give the message that you are angry not assertive (McCabe and Timmins, 2003).

However, while using assertive behaviour as a nurse is recommended (Hargie 2011), there are barriers in the workplace that prevent the use of assertive skills. Previous research (Poroch and McIntosh 1995) identified some of these barriers. These included

- A lack of knowledge about personal/professional rights.
- Concern about what others will think about one's behaviour.
- Anxiety due to a lack of confidence.
- Poor self-esteem.

Nurses appear to have an overriding concern with how others, the public and other health professionals view assertive behaviour among nurses. Assertive behaviour may conflict with the expectations of behaviour of a nice caring nurse (Valentine 1995; Percival 2001). Percival (2001) suggested that nurses have to live up to their public image of being 'nice' people, which militates against the use of assertive behaviour. Nice people usually accommodate and facilitate others rather than asserting their own rights (Percival 2001).

Research of nurses' use of assertive behaviour found that assertiveness is sometimes considered a negative behaviour

(Timmins and McCabe 2005). Nurses who use assertive behaviour are regarded as 'trouble makers' and 'cheeky'. Factors that prevented nurses being assertive were described as:

- nursing management,
- a fear of reprisal, and
- a fear of negative response from colleagues.

Nurses being assertive often left nurses feeling isolated and unsupported. 'Being assertive is often viewed as being a "trouble maker" ... It is less stressful not to assert oneself, and come in, do a day's work and go home' (Timmins and McCabe 2005: 38).

Poroch and McIntosh (1995) found that nurses feared rejection and isolation by colleagues if they used assertive, uncaring behaviour. The highest-ranking barrier to assertive behaviour in this group of nurses was the belief that it was an uncaring behaviour. McCartan (2001) reported a 'moderate' tendency for nurses to use assertion skills. Timmins and McCabe (2005) noted that few nurses in their study had received assertiveness education and many respondents cited a lack of knowledge as a barrier to using skills. In this study, managers emerged as a main barrier to using assertive skills (Timmins and McCabe 2005). In addition, the workplace atmosphere either served as a barrier or facilitated assertive behaviour.

An interesting finding from Timmins and McCabe's (2005) study was that respondents cited responsibility to the patient as a primary facilitator of their assertive behaviour. Clearly, from these practicing clinicians' perspective, assertiveness is a requirement of patient care. This corresponds with the increasing role of nurses as a patient advocate. This also congruent with Balzer-Riley's (2011) suggestion that assertiveness is a fundamental component of communication within the nurse–patient interaction and also of the therapeutic nurse–patient relationship. In the opening lines of the text *Communication in Nursing* (2011: ix) Balzer-Riley suggests that the book was designed to help nurses to 'be assertive to ask the right questions and make their voices heard. Nurses must be assertive to communicate their own needs and be prepared to assert themselves to ensure balance in their lives. Without such balance, the high stress environment may diminish nurses' effectiveness' thus suggesting that assertiveness is a fundamental component of effective nursing practice. Indeed, a third of the book is devoted to the topic of assertiveness. This emphasis on assertiveness is both novel and unique within the nursing literature. In some texts a chapter may be devoted to the topic, in others it is not discussed. Given the deficit in assertive behaviour by nurses (Timmins and McCabe 2005) together with the suggestion by nurses that their assertive behaviour was as a direct response to patient advocacy, we support Balzer-Riley's (2011) notion of the importance and centrality of assertiveness within the therapeutic nurse–patient relationship.

Registered nurses adhere to rigorous guidelines and codes and are called to account for actions. Contemporary nursing is set in a context of evidence-based practice. Nursing is continuously expanding its knowledge base through research and ongoing professional development to maintain competence. Nursing roles are expanding to increase specialist knowledge and skills. The requirement for continued education for registration requirements and the increasing repertoire of evidence-based nursing interventions both indicate a highly organized professional group. However, there are factors extrinsic to nursing that not only influence their perceived professional status but may also cause conflict. Their position within the hospital healthcare team can positively or negatively affect these perceptions.

Nurses have extensive social, legal, ethical and professional accountability. All of these aspects are quite separate in their definition but form complex interplay that informs nurses' day-to-day practice. There is also extensive legal accountability that recognizes nurses' authority and liability in practice. This responsibility is pervasive, and not straightforward. Carrying out the orders of other professional groups has inherent liability for nurses involved. The latter can results in ethical dilemmas and conflicts, not always experienced by professional groups with greater autonomy. Arnold and Underman Boggs (2011) suggest that it is these ethical dilemmas that cause some conflict for nurses. In Dowling et al.'s (2000) case study for example, nurses refused to deliver inappropriate orders. The doctors opposed their views. The nurses had to embark on a formal procedure route to raise their concerns, which were upheld. These situations are not uncommon for nurses who often risk isolation and retaliation, in the name of accountably, who may ultimately become 'whistleblowers' and risk job loss, if not supported in the practice setting (Brechin 2000).

It can also be difficult for nurses to behave assertively when they are working in high-pressure environments that cause stress (Balzer-Riley 2011). This is important to recognize within the healthcare setting. Patients and families often experience stress in this context, therefore an expectation that these persons would communicate assertively is unrealistic. While verbal and physical abuse is clearly intolerable in these settings, it is the nurse's responsibility to react appropriately where service users present with aggressive, passive or manipulative behaviour. The nurse, who ultimately holds responsibility for the communication, is in a better position, due to their lack of direct attachment and emotional involvement with recipients of care, to reflect maturely and consider the situation and choose an appropriate response.

Consider the nurse working in Accident and Emergency, where people typically wait for many hours to be seen by a doctor.

Example

When passing by the long queue she is approached by a person who is not happy waiting in the queue. Adopting a defensive response by saying 'we are a very busy department, you know, and if more people attended their GP it wouldn't be half as bad' may spark aggression in the person or may simply cause hurt and embarrassment. Whereas an assertive approach 'I understand how frustrating that must be for you, is there anything I can do to help?', not only reduces the risk of bad feelings and reactions from the person waiting, but also allows open communication to begin, that is not focused on the nurse's problems but is more patient/person centred.

It may well be that making a quick telephone call, or other simple solutions may ease the person's suffering in this case. Indeed clear information about the waiting times may also be useful, rather than a waiting time that is indefinite.

A relative, for example, who approaches the nurses' station in Accident and Emergency stands close to and above the level of nurse, shouts, pointing her finger 'my mother has been waiting for hours here and she is starving, can't I feed her something?'. An assertive response would include asking the relative to sit down, or standing to assume the same height. Then reflecting back the question 'you say that your mother has been waiting quite a while now, I am sorry that this is becoming difficult for her. Tell me a little more information and I will look into this for you'. Allowing the person to express her feelings in this regard, would allow some of the pent up aggression to abate. By remaining calm, and managing your own responses you can actually prevent conflict in the healthcare situation (Arnold and Underman Boggs 2011). Arnold and Underman Boggs (2011: 277) suggest that communication is the key to diffusing conflict situations: 'Give your undivided extra attention to a client or visitor whom you identify as potentially becoming aggressive'.

By maintaining eye contact, speaking in a quiet/normal voice in conjunction with the previous sentence the nurse encourages a more assertive response. In this case the reason for the outburst related to the relative's upset and feelings of anxiety and powerlessness related her mother's illness. The relative's frustration that had been redirected at the nursing staff emerged from her emotional reaction to her mother's illness. Once assertiveness skills were used, open person-centred communication allowed the relative to share many of these feelings. You might be able to let the family know how much longer they are likely to wait, confirm whether or not restriction of food is required, and perhaps offer something by way of comfort such as a separate room. Open honest communication is very valuable in these situations as it is often the not knowing that causes frustration. Assertiveness is often discussed synonymously with 'rights'. Commonly known as assertive rights further details are provided in Figure 6.2.

- I have the right to express my own feelings and opinions
- I have the right to state my own needs and set my own priorities as a person, independent of any roles that I may assume in life
- I have the right to be treated with respect as an intelligent, capable and equal human being
- I have the right to say 'no' or 'yes' for myself
- I have the right to make mistakes – and be responsible for them
- I have the right to change my mind
- I have the right to say 'I don't understand' and to ask for more information
- I have the right to ask for what I want
- I have the right to decline responsibility for other peoples problems
- I have the right to deal with people without being dependent on them for approval

Figure 6.2 Assertive rights

Source: McCabe, C. and Timmins, F. Teaching assertiveness to undergraduate nursing students, *Nurse Education in Practice* 3,1(2003) 30–42. Reproduced with kind permission from Elsevier Ltd

Although not implicit in Figure 6.2, assertiveness is also based on the premise that the other person within the interaction also has equal rights. From the earlier example, the nurse could have expressed her feelings thus: 'I feel very sad that your mum is becoming so uncomfortable, let me investigate this further for you'. One of the key aspects of assertive behaviour is that although exerting rights may be an expression of personal belief and opinion it does not actually confer those rights. For example, the right for you to make mistakes cannot be imposed on others. You cannot insist that others give you the right to make mistakes. Knowing and understanding your rights enables you to understand and have confidence in your basic human rights in a situation. However, attaining those rights is not the goal of the assertive communication but rather the expression of these. Bearing in mind however assertiveness behaviour may not be appropriate in all situations. If you are trying out assertiveness for the first time, for example, it might be best to try out these new techniques in a relatively safe environment by practising in front of a mirror or by returning a item to a shop, rather than keeping your first attempts for contentious issues or conflict situations in the clinical area, where your skills may require more practice.

Assertive behaviour is also described as a person giving expression to their rights, thoughts and feelings without denying the rights of others (Alberti and Emmons, 1986). Taylor (1989) suggested that within conflict one of the most common situations that involve assertiveness skills are where perceptions of the situation of the parties involved are quite different. Negotiating understanding is important. Taylor (1989) suggested that the benefits of using assertiveness in the management of conflict are: improved relationships, improved trust and openness, an increase in satisfaction and an improvement in decision-making. Taylor (1989: 5) suggested that assertion was 'about making oneself visible to others, standing up for oneself, if you like, in a way that seeks recognition and acknowledgement rather than insists upon being given in to'.

Taylor further distinguishes the 'assertive response' as combining the four Cs: clarity of communication, congruence of response, consistency about the issue and collaboration –inviting the other person to engage in this issue. Congruence is the 'match between what you say and what you do, what you say and how you feel', incongruence he suggests may be picked up by others and may reduce the impact of your attempts at assertiveness. Clarity involves stating a point simply, identifying the issues and sticking to it. It may mean repeating the point again and again.

Conclusion

Conflict is regarded as a natural part of the clinical environment. It can occur: within and between nurses; between nurses and other healthcare professionals; and between nurses, patients and patient's families. Nurses are often required to deal with conflict in the workplace. Resolving conflict requires identification of the conflict issues and the seeking of appropriate ways to address it. As a professional nurse it is important to deal with conflict rather than attempting to avoid it. One way of doing this is by developing assertiveness skills.

Nurses should use self-development to improve their conflict resolution skills. Assertiveness involves using specific responses to situations whereby the needs of all parties are considered equally. While barriers to using assertive skills in the clinical area may exist, nurses consider these important tools in patient advocacy. Clearly enticing or exacerbating aggressive reactions through poor communication skills in the practice setting is contrary to effective nursing practice, and while nurses' concern about their public image may seem to negate using assertive skills, ultimately this is one of the best ways to deal effectively with, reduce and resolve conflict in the healthcare situations. Assertive behaviour may conflict with the expectations of behaviour of a 'nice caring nurse'. Communication is the key to diffusing conflict situations. Patient-centred communication requires a continuing awareness by nurses, as individuals, of their contribution to interactions that they have with patients, relatives, friends, other healthcare professionals and healthcare staff. Therefore, the use by nurses of behaviours other than assertive behaviour with these consumers of healthcare limits the chance of the communication being truly patient-centred.

Key points

▶ Assertive behaviour and negotiation skills are regarded as essential skills in allowing nurses to be autonomous practitioners within a multidisciplinary team.

▶ Conflict is inevitable in an environment where many healthcare disciplines work together. It can be positive but if it is not managed appropriately it can become negative and destructive.

▶ Collaboration is the most effective response in assertiveness because it facilitates the development of mutually satisfying solutions.

▶ Hierarchical healthcare structures and workplace atmospheres are often not only a cause of conflict but also prevent conflict from being managed successfully and positively.

7 Collaborative Communication

Introduction

Throughout this textbook, many of the chapters refer to the importance of healthcare professionals working together and how good communication skills are essential to this. This chapter outlines the reasons why collaborative communication and interprofessional working are so important. It explores the process and the elements that make it successful and the barriers that obstruct it. You may find it useful to revise Chapters 4, 5 and 6 before you read this chapter as collaborative communication requires the use of the many skills and behaviours discussed in these chapters.

The provision of high-quality and patient-centred health care is dependent on all healthcare professions working collaboratively (Wright and Brajtman 2011). This approach is expected by governments and regulatory bodies for the development, implementation and evaluation of healthcare policy and services at local, national and international levels. However, it seems that this approach remains inspirational rather than reality. The absence of interprofessional collaborative working between doctors, nurses or hospital managers for example, is commonly cited as the main cause of fragmented and task-oriented care and may be the cause of up to 70 per cent of reported adverse incidents (Fewster-Thuente and Velsor-Friedrich 2008; Dingley et al. 2008). Furthermore multidisciplinary working rather than interprofessional collaboration does not acknowledge the multidimensional nature of what it is to be an individual and that people should not be regarded as composites of systems or parts (Francis 2010). Collaborative communication and systems facilitate healthcare professionals, managers and patients working together towards the common goal of patient-centred care rather than working separately.

Interprofessional, collaborative practice requires that all healthcare professionals who are involved come together with the patient to develop, implement and evaluate a plan of care. It is not the common current multidisciplinary approach where the different professions assess, plan and evaluate the care of the patient independent of both the patient and other professions (Orchard 2010).

Process of collaborative communication

The process of collaboration requires mutual understanding and respect, articulated and agreed shared goals and awareness and mutual protection of each group's roles and boundaries. In order for collaborative communication to be facilitated it needs to be supported by systems embedded in the larger organizational structure (McCabe 2010). Examples of this include interventions such as:

- a standardized communication tool such as the SBAR,
- an early warning score or escalation process,
- daily multiprofessional patient-centred rounds that include completion of a daily goals sheet, and
- discussions during each shift.

The communication tool known as SBAR (Situation, Background, Assessment, Recommendation) is a useful framework developed for the purpose of facilitating collaborative communication between healthcare professionals (Permanente 2012). Dingley et al. (2008) report that the introduction of such collaborative working strategies is effective and enhances interprofessional communication. However, other studies report that communication tools and strategies alone do not significantly improve collaborative communication between healthcare professionals. They report that collaborative communication education is fundamental to the success of introducing such strategies as it provides information about why such strategies are necessary, different communication styles and potential outcomes (Thompson et al. 2011; Beckett and Kipnis 2009). This in turn increases staff 'buy in' into the commitment to change to improve their communication skills. This tool has been extended to ISBAR (Introduction/Identify, Situation, Background, Assessment, Recommendation) (Beckett and Kipnis 2009).

Example

You are a newly qualified staff nurse and find it difficult to communicate clearly with some of the senior staff, for example, doctors, nurses and administrators. They generally seem irritated when you try to make a request or give handover and it is causing you considerable stress.

Your hospital has recently introduced an early warning score system that includes the communication tool ISBAR and after receiving some education about collaborative communication, you are determined to use it to help improve your personal communication skills. An opportunity arises when you are on an evening shift and at 7 p.m. the condition of one of your patients begins to deteriorate. The doctor on call is one that you have found it particularly difficult to communicate with in the past as he does not hide his impatience and frustration. However, you decide to proceed with using the ISBAR tool and have it written on the handover notes that you keep in your pocket.

Introduction/Identify

Hi Mike, this is Jane from ward 2. I am the staff nurse looking after Mr X

Situation

He has a pyrexia of 38.5, his pulse rate is 98, his respirations are 22 per minute and his oxygen saturation level is 95 on room air.

Background

Mr X is 22 years old, had surgery last night following a ruptured appendix and is on morphine for pain management, IV fluids and IV antibiotics. He does not have any other medical/surgical history and is not on any other medication.

Assessment
He has an early warning score of 6. This afternoon his condition deteriorated with an increase in his respiratory rate and pulse rate and a drop in his O_2 saturation levels. His temperature has increased also from 38 at 4 p.m. this afternoon to 38.5. His urinary catheter has drained 100mls of concentrated in the past 3 hours. The surgical wound is slightly inflamed but there is no exudate.

Recommendation
I think that you need to review this patient as soon as possible and take arterial blood gases. In the meantime I will take bloods for FBC, U+E and culture, commence oxygen therapy and increase the rate of IV fluids if you are in agreement.

Doctor's response
Yes that's fine, I'll be there in 5 minutes (tone is matter-of-fact, not irritated or impatient).

After this interaction, it is clear to you that ISBAR has helped you to communicate clearly and collaboratively and you feel more confident about working with other professionals in the future.

An important point to note from this scenario is Jane's awareness of her own communication deficits and her commitment and willingness to use new and challenging strategies that will, ultimately, help her to improve. The ISBAR tool is not just for use in nurse-doctor communication, it is relevant in all communication, even with patients or non health care personnel. It provides a framework that allows the user to impart relevant information in a succinct, objective manner. Remember that non-verbal communication is equally important when using tools such as ISBAR.

Other more formal modes of interprofessional collaboration exist, for example, in shared decision making practice where patient/family and the relevant members of the multidisciplinary healthcare team meet to evaluate care and discuss further treatment. These meetings are called family conferences or patient case meetings and nurses are required to contribute significantly in order to advocate for patients and ensure that the patient receives optimal care.

Example

Peter is a 72 year old man who had a stroke and has been in hospital for three weeks. He has left side weakness but is beginning to mobilize with assistance. He lives alone with a pet dog that has been cared for by a neighbour since he became ill. Peter has one son who lives with his family 200 km away in another town. He phones his father once a week but only comes to see him every 3–4 months. A family conference has been arranged to develop a plan for the future treatment and needs of Peter in preparation for discharge.

The ward manager, staff nurse (John who has just qualified and has cared for Peter over the past three weeks), the doctor, physiotherapist, occupational therapist and dietician attend the conference along with Peter and his son. During the conference the doctor and physiotherapist agree that Peter has a significant disability as a result of the stroke and will need a great deal of support to live independently. They suggest that Peter would benefit from living in a residential care setting. The ward manager agrees and recommends a local nursing home to Peter's son who asks for contact details for the home. Peter asks if it is not possible for to return home but his son and the healthcare team feel that he would not be safe and needs support. Peter appears to agree and nods his head. As the meeting is coming to an end it seems that Peter will be discharged to the nursing home when arrangements have been made but John (his staff nurse) speaks with a nervous and quiet voice saying that Peter has told him previously that although he does not want to be a burden to anyone, he does not want to live in a nursing home either. When Peter's son points out that he lives so far away and would not be able to help out, John says that he has met Peter's neighbour on a few occasions when she has visited Peter and that she would be happy to become his carer. Peter's son is very interested to hear this and says that he will speak to the neighbour because he would rather his father live at home if that was his wish as long as he was safe. The team agree that another family conference would take place one week later and Peter's discharge plan could be finalized then. John was relieved that he spoke up even though he found it difficult in front of so many people.

Interprofessional collaboration at management level requires nurses to contribute in group settings usually at a meeting where different professions are represented. The ISBAR communication tool in conjunction with communication skills such as assertiveness, persuasion and negotiation are key skills required at this level. However, it is important to note that the person chairing such committees will be the primary influence on how collaborative the process is. The chair is usually a manager who could be from a nursing, medical or administrative background but that is not as important as whether or not they value, support and facilitate interprofessional collaborative communication.

Barriers to successful collaborative communication

The barriers to successful collaborative communication occur at many different levels, for example, hierarchical approaches to the management of healthcare institutions and services may not encourage, support or facilitate different disciplines working together towards a common goal. The culture is more representative of a multidisdiplinary approach with a top-down management style rather than an open collaborative interprofessional patient-centred focus. The reason for this is probably because it is sometimes regarded as an idealistic and time-consuming strategy (DeVito 2011). Organizational and/or personal commitment to communicating collaboratively with colleagues will require additional time. This is not excessive and with the provision of safer and more patient-centred care and services, the professional and organizational benefits of providing a higher standard of care considerably outweigh the time required.

Historical power imbalances exist between the professions with each believing that collaborative working will diminish their profession in some way or that they are more important than all other professions and administrators who contribute to patient care and, therefore, should be listened to have the final say. Interestingly Orchard (2010: 254) proposes that it is not necessarily other professions that prevent nurses from working collaboratively, it is nurses themselves who 'remove themselves and remain persistent isolationists from moving in the collaborative practice direction' thus allowing other professions to appear to contribute more significantly to patient care and also policy development.

Success at competition for resources has always been a source of power in healthcare services and it is also perceived that the profession that receives the most resources, which translates into funding for services, equipment and staff is the most important. However, the current focus on healthcare funding following the patient rather than the professions or service will play a significant role in removing this as a barrier to interprofessional working.

A key barrier to collaborative communication in nursing is the lack of competence in articulating what nursing is and how it contributes in terms of nursing knowledge and skill to the provision of patient-centred care Orchard (2010). It is essential that all professions and disciplines involved articulate their role because not only does it clarify what each profession contributes, it also establishes role boundaries. This is reassuring for all involved in collaborative working and will assist in minimizing conflict (Reber et al. 2011).

Successful collaborative communication

In order to develop the necessary communication skills required for working collaboratively with other professions and administrators as equal contributors in the provision of true patient-centred care requires specific focus and commitment outside normal working hours (Reeves 2009).

Specific communication skills required by individuals for interprofessional collaborative working include assertiveness, negotiation and openness underpinned by knowledge, a positive attitude and a willingness to work with other disciplines.

Each chapter in this book has presented the communication skills required to communicate effectively, positively and in a patient-centred way. The verbal and non-verbal skills of listening, questioning and paraphrasing are key components of collaborative communication. These skills are used in conjunction with communication behaviours such as assertiveness and all are influenced by your personal values, belief about yourself as a person, as a nurse and your perceived role as an equal member of an interdisciplinary collaborative team. Using these skills to develop or enhance your ability to communicate collaboratively is essential to demonstrate a willingness to work collaboratively with other professions and patients. Nadzam (2009: 187) proposes the following communication behaviours and actions as a means of facilitating one-to-one successful collaborative working.

- Address the physician by name.
- Have patient information and the chart readily available.
- Clearly express any concern about the patient and the reason for that concern.
- Suggest a follow-up plan.
- Focus on the patient problem, not extenuating circumstances.
- Be professional, not aggressive.
- Continue to monitor the patient problem until it has been resolved.

This list encompasses many of the ISBAR tool elements and also recognizes the personal contribution that individuals make to any interaction and in ensuring that the communication behaviours they use are positive and objective. One of the reasons that collaborative communication can be difficult is because it requires that those involved listen actively and are mutually respectful of each other's role, contribution and views.

As discussed in Chapter 4, developing new communication skills or behaviours is not easy. It requires attention and practice over time. Gardner (2005) describes 10 personal attributes that will help you develop successful interpersonal collaborative skills.

1. Self awareness.
2. Accept, value and use diversity to produce collaborative outcomes.
3. Develop positive conflict resolution skills and learn to use conflict as a tool for ideas and learning.
4. Develop good negotiation skills that recognize and value your contribution as an equal member of the healthcare team to the provision of patient-centred care.
5. Ensure that you are clinically competent, cooperative and flexible in work practices.
6. Recognize that collaboration is a continuous process.
7. Make your presence felt at multidisciplinary forums by contributing in a confident, knowledgeable and collegial manner that demonstrates respect for all other professionals involved.
8. Appreciate that collaboration often occurs spontaneously and without conscious thought.
9. Always be reflective and learn from collaborative experiences with other professionals – it is good to seek feedback and discuss decision-making processes.
10. Be aware that collaboration is not always necessary for all decisions.

In order to be successful and effective at collaborating and minimize conflict, the skills of persuasion and negotiation are very important. This is as relevant when communicating with patients and their families about appropriate treatments and plans for care as it is with other healthcare professionals and administrators.

Persuasion

Persuasion is our ability to influence others to do what we want and in turn we can be persuaded by others. It happens during formal and informal interactions between people. Hargie (2011) describes four elements of persuasion;

1. Resistance – persuasion is required only if resistance is present.
2. Conscious awareness – manipulation of face-to-face communication to convince others to do what you want.
3. Direction – persuasion is a one way process with one person/group trying to persuade another.
4. Success – if it was not successful then persuasion did not happen.

As most of us are aware our attempts are sometime successful but not always. Possible outcomes of persuasion include instant success in the form of attitudinal, behavioural or value change, increased resistance to persuasion attempts, no change or delayed success that can happen after the initial attempt to persuade. Factors that can help or hinder attempts to persuade others include:

Relationship – having a positive, close relationship or commonalities with those we are trying to persuade will help our chances of success as those we are trying to persuade will be more trusting. This is enhanced by the use of good verbal and non-verbal communication skills.

Attractiveness – physical and social attractiveness also increases success when persuading others.

Humour – appropriate, moderate amounts of humour are also helpful in being persuasive.

Narratives – tell stories about how others have been persuaded and the benefits it brought to them. This is a particularly useful strategy in healthcare, for example, when a nurse is encouraging someone to commence and maintain an exercise regimen following hip replacement surgery. Stories about other patient's successful recovery can be inspiring for patients who are reluctant or are experiencing difficulties in mobilizing.

Power – those who are perceived to have power tend to be more successful as persuading others to do what they want.

Expertise – it is important that those you are trying to persuade are aware of your knowledge and expertise. This enhances your credibility and increases the chances of bringing about the changes you want.

Example: nurse–patient interaction

Ann works as a staff nurse on a medical ward and is talking to a patient about the link between smoking and the recent diagnosis of mild chronic obstructive pulmonary disease (COPD) that the patient has received.

Patient: Is there anything I can do to stop the COPD from getting worse, I am only 60 years of age and I do not want this to stop me from dancing and socializing with my friends.

Nurse: Yes there are definite actions that you can take and actually dancing is an activity that you should maintain as exercise is very important for managing COPD. I know someone who is much worse than you and needs oxygen all the time but she still dances twice a week.

Nurse: Have you thought about how you are going to stop smoking?

Patient: No but I suppose it's something I'll have to do at some stage. It's great that it won't affect my dancing, I really enjoy it and it's a great way to meet all my friends.

Nurse: I think that if you stop smoking now it will help more than anything. I have worked with people with COPD for 10 years and although they find it difficult, they all say that it was worth it and helped to stop the COPD from getting worse.

Patient: I've tried to stop smoking before but I never lasted longer than 3 weeks so I don't think I could do it now either.

Nurse: I know it's a big change but you could still do everything else that you like doing and it would mean that your condition won't get worse. How about giving up the smoking altogether and taking up more dancing (laughing)!

Patient: I'd like more dancing, I'm quite good actually (smiling). When I was younger I used to teach it. I suppose you are right about the smoking but I'm not sure …

Nurse: Would you like to talk to someone about it? I can get the nurse specialist to come and see you later today and we can take it from there.

Patient: Yes I think that is a good idea because otherwise I might not do anything about it

This scenario demonstrates a number of the important elements of persuasion such as humour, expertise and having a positive relationship with the patient.

The success of using persuasion in nursing, for example, when collaborating with a patient in devising a plan of care and trying to agree on the responsibilities of the nurse and the patient in the partnership it essential that the nurse takes the time to get to know the patient. This means that efforts to persuade are tailored to the individual, therefore, therefore the patient feels more in control and is more likely to make behavioural or attitudinal changes. If patients feel that they are not being listened to or if they are being forced into accepting something that they do not understand or agree with, they are more likely to reject attempts at persuasion (Rains and Turner 2007).

Negotiation

As we have seen in Chapter 6 conflict is an integral part of life and is particularly so when working in an environment where interaction with other healthcare and non-healthcare professionals, patients and their families is a predominant part of the day-to-day job. It is not surprising that negotiation is a very valuable and essential communication skill. There are many ways to describe negotiation but generally speaking certain elements need to exist in order for negotiation to take place. These elements are: a degree of disagreement or resistance from one or both parties; and a mutual interest in an exchange of service, goods, information, time or money that will have some benefit for both. Unlike persuasion it is a two-way process and can be a formal or informal, simple or complex, for example, arranging time-off around holiday time can take some skilful negotiation with colleagues to get reach an agreement that everyone is happy with. A more formal and complex type of negotiation could be organizing community care services for a patient who has multiple needs and whose family is only able to provided limited care.

Negotiation is regarded as an essential communication strategy for nurses in ensuring patient participation in the provision of patient-centred care. Sahlsten et al. (2007) suggest that negotiation in nursing is an exchange, cooperation and bargaining to find common ground between firmly different purposes. It will not be successful or beneficial to all parties with knowledge or understanding and underpinned by mutual respect. It is an essential ingredient for successful collaboration.

Example: nurse–patient negotiation
In this scenario the patient is 24 hours post appendectomy and has been reluctant to mobilize. The nurse needs to ensure that she mobilizes as soon as possible.

Nurse: Good Morning Susan, are you ready to get up yet?

Susan: No, I'm tired and it really hurts when I move.

Nurse: Ok, well how about if I get some analgesia for you straight away and while we are waiting for that to take effect, I'll see to the patient in the room next door?

Susan: That would be great, thanks. I know I need to get out of bed but right now I just don't feel able to and I think the medication will help.

Example: nurse–doctor negotiation
In this scenario the nurse is concerned because they are expecting two admissions from the emergency department but patients who are due to go home have not yet been discharged by the doctor.

Nurse: Hello Mike, its Catherine calling from Ward 3. We are expecting two admissions from the emergency department so will you come up to discharge Mr. X and Mrs. Y, they are probably ready to go home today. You need to review their wounds before they go and write their prescriptions.

Doctor: I am just heading into theatre so I won't be able to go to the ward for at least another hour.

Nurse: The emergency department is under considerable pressure to admit patients, and I have all the documents ready for discharging Mr. X and Mrs. Y. If you come up to the ward straightaway I don't think it will take you long, I have had a look at their wounds and they are healing well. All you will need to do is write the prescriptions.

Doctor: I do not have time to do this right now.

Nurse: I understand that you are busy but if you can discharge these two patients now, it would help us on this ward and the emergency department a great deal. Their families are already here with them so they will be able to leave as soon as you are finished.

Doctor: Ok, I'll be there in straightaway

The scenario demonstrates everyday informal negotiation skills that nurses use to help patients and professional colleagues that also allow them to work efficiently and effectively.

Key points

▶ The unique role of the nurse can only be achieved through nurses working collaboratively with other healthcare disciplines. Collaboration is not a communication behaviour that nurses (or other healthcare professionals) are renowned for but it is a communication skill that is essential if nurses are to care for patients in a therapeutic and patient-centred way.

▶ The process of collaboration requires a mutual understanding and respect by all involved, articulated and agreed shared goals, awareness and mutual protection of each groups roles and boundaries.

▶ Barriers to successful interprofessional collaborative communication in healthcare include a perpetuating hierarchical organization structure that supports historical power imbalances between the professions and hospital managers. In nursing alone the greatest barrier is its inability to articulate what nursing is and its unique contribution to the provision of patient-centred care.

▶ Successful interprofessional collaborative communication requires attention, commitment and support structures from an organizational and individual perspective. It is based on good verbal and non-verbal communication, assertive behaviour and self-awareness.

▶ The skills of persuasion and negotiation are fundamental to ensuring successful collaboration in nursing and are particularly useful in minimizing conflict and maintaining a focus on an interdisciplinary approach to patient-centred care.

8 Communicating in Difficult Situations

Introduction

Some situations are perceived by students as 'difficult' due to the emotional content, perceived lack of communication ability and cultural differences. These situations pose a significant challenge for personal and professional development. They can involve a combination of interactions with patients, their relatives and colleagues. Learning to communicate in an effective and patient- or person-centred way in these situations is essential for developing confidence and positive relationships. However, students often feel that although the theory delivered in class situations is relevant, it does not prepare them for the reality of dealing with these situations. In this chapter we aim to help students meet these challenges by providing theory in relation to dealing with issues such as breaking bad news, anxiety, hostility and cultural differences. In conjunction with this theory we will demonstrate to students that by learning to manage themselves in difficult situations, rather than trying to manage others who may be emotionally distressed or poor communicators themselves, a much more positive and patient- or person-centred outcome can be achieved. Although this chapter will deal specifically with the difficult issues associated with breaking bad news, cultural issues and anxiety and hostility, it is important to acknowledge that the situations that individuals perceive as difficult vary greatly. This is primarily because of their existing communication skills, their level of self-confidence and their past experiences in relation to a particular situation, for example, some nurses may find it more difficult to approach their manager to request study leave or annual leave than helping a patient who has received bad news or helping a recently bereaved family.

If nurses perceive that they do not have the communication skills needed to communicate effectively in 'difficult' situations they may avoid them or they may communicate in a negative or unhelpful way. This can have an adverse affect on a nurse's level of confidence and overall professional development. Also if a nurse avoids dealing with very emotive situations, patients can feel very lonely and isolated because the nurse does not acknowledge or talk about what is happening to the patient. It is therefore essential that the communication skills required to deal successfully and appropriately with difficult situations are recognized, developed and practiced by nurses.

One of the most effective learning opportunities for students in seeing how certain communication skills can help in difficult situations is to identify a role model. Identify a nurse who is known to be a good communicator, that is, kind, sympathetic, non-judgmental, open and friendly. With these characteristics and experience she will probably also be empathetic. You can usually identify these nurses from your own experiences with them or through observing how they tend to have very positive relationships with patients and colleagues. If a nurse is kind, supportive and helpful towards students, then it is probably fair to say that they are the same towards patients and their colleagues and is, therefore, a good role model. In addition to using a good or positive role model it is also helpful to identify a nurse whose communication skills are not as positive and observe how poor communication skills impact on the nurse–patient relationship and patient care generally.

Managing yourself in difficult situations

As mentioned earlier, it is important that a nurse learns to manage himself/herself in difficult situations. If they are unable to do this or are not aware of their skills and behaviours then they will find it difficult to build confidence in approaching and dealing with difficult situations effectively. This section talks about the need to know yourself and the assumptions, values, beliefs and attitudes that you hold that influence your approach toward people both socially and in your work. If you feel this is an aspect of yourself that you have not thought much about then it might be beneficial for you to read Chapter 10, which deals with the role of self-concept, self-awareness and self-esteem in personal and professional development before completing this chapter. By identifying our hidden assumptions, values, beliefs and attitudes it is possible to interpret situations that we perceive to be difficult in a more accurate way. When this happens we take more patient-centred and helpful action. Our reaction to situations that were previously perceived as difficult is now more manageable and less stressful.

Example

A nurse is in the process of admitting a very elderly lady to an acute medical ward. The lady appears to be confused, is agitated and has a high temperature. Her personal hygiene is very poor and she is very thin. Her next of kin is documented as her daughter who lives with her and brought her to hospital. She has gone home to bring in some clothes, shoes and other personal belongings for her mother. The nurse discusses this patient with a nursing colleague and voices her annoyance with the lady's daughter because the lady is so physically unwell and unkempt. The nurse's irritation grows as it takes a number of hours for the patient's daughter to return to the hospital with her mother's belongings. When the nurse enters the patient's room she sees the daughter sitting in a chair beside her mother's bed. With an irritated tone and loud voice the nurse asks the daughter to give her some details for the nursing notes regarding her mother's illness and medical history. The daughter begins to tell the nurse how her father, the patient's husband, died four weeks previously and he was the main carer for her mother who had been in bad health for a number of years. The nurse's facial expression shows her further irritation as her continuous cold tone asks why the patient's condition deteriorated so rapidly and why she did not come to hospital sooner. The daughter then becomes upset and tells the nurse that she herself has poor health and although she tried to look after her mother she could not manage. When the nurse asks her why she could not manage the daughter becomes even more distressed and shows her hands and wrists that are grossly deformed as a result of chronic arthritis. The nurse is immediately sympathetic and her attitude towards the patient and her mother changes to a more sensitive and supportive approach.

This example describes how ordinary everyday events at work can become stressful or negative. This example highlights how hidden assumptions can make interpretations of situations inaccurate and reactions negative. It also supports the discussion in Chapter 4 that asking the questions starting with 'why' can be judgmental and questions using 'what' or 'how' can provide more specific, focused questions that are less judgmental or difficult to answer. The thing about our assumptions, values, beliefs and attitudes is that they exist sometimes within our consciousness but often outside our consciousness. What we need to do to manage ourselves in difficult situations is to identify them so that we can change or ignore our assumptions, values, beliefs and attitudes in order to focus on the needs of patients in many different contexts.

Anxiety also plays a key role in how a nurse communicates with a patient and can make some situations difficult for both the nurse and the patient. Anxiety is an emotional response that represents feelings of discomfort, insecurity or fear. It generally manifests physically as nausea or sweating and in person's behaviour (Moser et al. 2003). The anxiety can be nurse related, patient related or both, for example, a nurse may be anxious about removing sutures from a wound because they may hurt the patient or they may not have much experience in removing sutures. Likewise the patient may be feeling anxious because they think the procedure will be painful. Anxiety can trigger hostile or angry responses in people because they are misinterpreting your words. They may not even be aware of their own anxiety and this can make the situation even more difficult and prevent effective communication. Every person whether it is a patient or family member experiences some level of anxiety when in hospital. This means that when communicating, nurses need to keep this in mind and understand that one person can be as anxious about having heart surgery as another person having a toe nail removed. An appreciation of this will help nurses communicate more appropriately and in a patient-centred way when helping patients to identify the possible causes of their anxiety. Kreigh and Perco (1983) refer to anxiety as mild, moderate or severe and describe the effect of anxiety on behaviour and ability to think clearly.

Mild anxiety – thinking and coping ability is enhanced and behaviours may include walking, humming, restlessness but focused when necessary. A nurse will experience this before carrying out a procedure for the first time, like catheterization or removing sutures.

Moderate anxiety – concentration and ability to think clearly is reduced and the person may not know what is making them anxious. They will appear tense and possibly agitated, angry or even withdrawn. At this level of anxiety they will respond well to support and guidance. This level of anxiety is apparent in patients and their relatives when on admission to hospital or just prior to surgery.

Severe anxiety – cannot think logically or coherently even with guidance. Behaviour is unfocused and possibly inappropriate. Response to support and guidance is not immediate. Referral to a psychologist or psychiatrist is recommended.

Example of how anxiety influences communication
A young woman is admitted to the emergency department following a road traffic accident. She has a concussion and minor facial lacerations. Shortly afterwards her father arrives in the department and spends some time with her. Then he leaves to go home to get some personal items for his daughter who needs to be admitted but returns to the department almost immediately to say that his car has been clamped by hospital parking attendants. He is very irate and the nurse finds it difficult to calm him down. He says that there were no parking places when he arrived and he had to park in a 'no parking' zone. His anxiety about his daughter meant that he felt that the only option was to park illegally. The nurse

understands this and asks the man to take a seat beside her while she phones the parking attendant. She explains the situation to the parking attendant who says that the clamp will be removed without charge but that the man will have to wait about 20 minutes. The man complains further when he hears this but the nurse uses this opportunity to talk to him about his daughter's accident and what treatment she will need. Eventually the man starts to tell the nurse about how scared he was driving to the hospital and not knowing what to expect and after a few minutes he thanks the nurse for helping him out and goes to spend more time with his daughter before the clamp is removed from his car.

The following points are useful for ensuring effective communication and helping patients deal with anxiety:

- Always appreciate that being admitted to hospital, regardless of the reason provokes anxiety in patients and their relatives.
- Actively address the concerns of the patient or relative. In the above example the nurse deals with the clamping issue before she addresses the main cause of the man's anxiety, which is his daughter and her injuries. Trying to reduce a persons' level of anxiety without dealing with their immediate concerns will be ineffective and may only heighten their anxiety.
- Ensure privacy when trying to reduce a patient's or relative's anxiety and let them know that you are genuinely concerned for them. Pull the curtains around the bed, sit if possible and look at the patient and relatives when they speak. Active listening is an essential skill in helping people deal with their anxiety. Be honest about the choices a person has or what the situation is and do not make promises you cannot keep. Speak slowly and repeat the main points if necessary. Just because you attempt to reduce a person's anxiety level, do not assume that they will respond positively. They may not be ready to talk but by checking on them and keeping them updated with information, patients and their relatives will

begin to trust the nurse and this will reduce their anxiety levels.

- Be aware of your own levels of anxiety. This will allow you to deal more effectively with the anxieties of others or help you realize that maybe you are not the best person to help. This is important because a key role in nursing is recognizing when a patient needs someone else to help them besides a nurse. A counsellor, psychologist or psychiatrist is often the most appropriate person to help a patient deal with moderate or severe levels of anxiety.

Breaking bad news

Nurses do not usually break bad news to patients directly but are generally, although not always, present when patients and their families are given bad news. A key role of the nurse is to clarify, explain and expand on what the doctor said. However, before we discuss how to do that it is essential to talk about what nurses expect to contribute to family, relatives and friends who have just lost a loved one or to a patient who has just heard that they have a terminal illness or will need to have a leg amputated. The role of the nurse in caring for patient is to provide physical or psychological comfort and support. However, when caring for a bereaved relative, nurses can find it difficult to see the results of their endeavours. Usually they never know if they made any difference to how that person coped when they heard the bad news. As nurses do not receive feedback from the bereaved person they may assume incorrectly that they did not help sufficiently and many therefore try to detach themselves from these situations. On a personal level nurses, especially if they have experienced a recent bereavement, can find it difficult. One thing that might help nurses communicate in a more patient-centred, sensitive and supportive way in a situation that they find very stressful themselves is to realize that they are not there to make the person feel better. This is probably the worst day of that person's life so to think that as a nurse they can make it better is very presumptuous and sets an unachievable goal. However, a nurse can help the person in a number of different ways. These include:

- Give the family as much time as they need – it can take a whole morning to help a family after ensuring that you have met their needs and given them all the information they need.
- Bring the person or family to a private area.
- Offer beverages.
- Stay with the family even if no one is talking. This does not mean that you are not needed. They may suddenly think of a question about how the person died or what happens next and if you are there to answer it will help them get through the day. It is always best not to talk too much. Silence may be difficult for the nurse but can be comforting for the bereaved because they will be lost in their own thoughts. They will talk if they want to and all the nurse needs to do is to listen. If as a nurse you have an intense need to talk it can result in you making a judgmental comment or unconsciously agreeing when a family member blames himself or herself.

Example

Wife: I last saw John (the dead person) when I brought him a cup of tea in the living room. He was watching TV and he said thanks when I put it down beside him. The phone rang then and it was Louise, our daughter and when I went back in to him, he wasn't breathing. That's when I called the ambulance.

Nurse: How long were you on the phone for?

Wife: About half an hour, perhaps if I had gone back in sooner??

Regardless of the reason for the nurse asking this question, it gave the woman feelings of guilt and added to her distress. The only time a nurse needs to talk is to answer questions asked and reassure the family and relatives in any way they can. Non-verbal communication is probably more effective in situations like this.

Bad news

Being present when a patient hears bad news can be upsetting for all involved. Sometimes the doctor and nurse will plan together how the patient will hear the news or the nurse may just be present when the doctor gives the patient the news but usually after the patient hears the news and some explanation about what will happen next, the doctor leaves the room. The nurse should remain with the patient to support them, clarify information and answer any questions they might have. Key principles apply to any situation where a patient hears bad news.

- The nurse needs to ensure that they have time to spend with the patient. Do not appear hurried or rushed, as this will make the patient feel that they are keeping you from something more important. Spending time with the patient may be immediately after they hear the news or shortly afterwards. Sometimes the patient might want to be left alone or with family when they hear bad news but it is important that the nurse returns in a specified amount of time to talk to the patient.
- Do not make assumptions about what information the patient wants. If you are unsure *ask the patient!* 'Hi John, would you like to talk about what the doctor told you?'
- Before giving any information ask the patient if they have any questions. This means that the information they receive is pertinent or important to them at that time. A number of visits may be required because the patient will need to have information repeated because people generally only retain 60 per cent of what they hear in normal situations and if they are very anxious they are likely to hear even less. They will also think of questions as they reflect on the news they received and try to make plans for the future when they are alone or discussing the news with their family.
- It is important to find out what the patient knows about their illness and the implications of the news they have heard. When this is established it is essential to determine what information the patient wants to hear. The only way to this is to talk to the patient and ask them to tell you what

they know. Follow their lead and observe their emotional behaviour as they do this. If a patient does not appear to have much information by asking them directly if they would like more information on their illness they will indicate very quickly how much information they want.

● If they request more information ask them if they would like to have a family member present. This can be reassuring for them and two people can remember more than one.

Even though information concerning a patient is confidential sometimes a doctor does not give the patient the bad news instead the next of kin and family are informed first. The family may then decide to tell the patient themselves or ask the doctor to tell them. Although legally and ethically, no one has the right to, occasionally the next of kin and family decide not to tell the patient the news because they feel that the patient would not want to hear the news. This is known as collusion and can create difficulties for nurses as they care for the patient as their physical condition deteriorates. The patient may ask the nurse why they are not getting better and because the nurse cannot explain what is happening to the patient, the patient can feel very confused and isolated. In order to prevent such scenarios the nurse can respond to a request not to tell the patient anything in a number of ways:

Example: Responding to a request to withhold bad news

Family member: Nurse the doctor has just told me and my family that John's cancer has spread and all they can offer is palliative care. We don't want John to know about this because it would only upset him make him lose hope.

Nurse: I understand that but as a nurse I think it is important to find out what John already knows or suspects about what is happening to him. He may not be saying anything because he is trying to protect all of you. Maybe if I talk to him and see if he knows anything and if he does maybe you should all get together and talk.

> *Family member*: And what if he doesn't seem to know anything?
>
> *Nurse*: In that case there may not be any need for you to talk at the moment, however, I should tell you that if he asks me anything about his illness, I cannot withhold information and will answer his questions truthfully.

Grief and bereavement

Death and dying is one particular area where students and newly qualified nurses find it difficult to use theory to inform their practice and probably for good reason. Theory related to bereavement and grief is usually centred on the work of theorists such as Kubler-Ross (1973), Engel (1972) and Lindemann (1944). Lindemann's (1944) theory emphasizes the immediate physical reaction that people experience when they hear bad news or a relative/friend dies. This response includes tightness in the throat, shortness of breath, sighing, feeling empty and a lack of muscle power. Intense emotional distress accompanies the physical response. Engel's (1972) theory describes the bereavement process in stages. These include:

1. shock, disbelief, denial;
2. developing awareness;
3. re-institution phase;
4. resolving the loss; and the
5. idealization phase.

Similarly Kubler-Ross's theory identifies five stages to the bereavement process. These include:

1. denial and isolation,
2. anger,
3. bargaining,
4. depression, and
5. acceptance.

Although perhaps relevant to some people's experiences of bereavement, the work of Kubler-Ross (1973) and others who refer to dealing with bereavement as a series of stages is increasingly criticized by social scientists. The stages are useful in that they comprise descriptions of a variety of emotional responses to bad news and bereavement; the use of the term 'stages' indicates that an individual progresses through each stage either sequentially or at some point in their grieving/bereavement process. Therefore, when a nurse witnesses a reaction that does not fit any of these descriptions, they can perceive it as abnormal. An example of this is when people from some cultures hear bad news or are bereaved they demonstrate their distress physically by throwing themselves on the floor or wailing. Other cultures, particularly western cultures exhibit a more restrained response to grief and bereavement. The following quote is from a woman talking about the death of her 11-week-old baby and demonstrates the typical response to grief and bereavement in western culture. 'I wanted to shout and scream – to tear my hair out – to keen. But I didn't. I behaved like a first-world woman and just cried until there was nothing left' (Anon. 1994). Harms' multidimensional model (2007) discussed in Chapter 1 provides an explanation as to why individuals may respond differently to similar situations. Being aware of this and not being judgmental will help the nurse manage their own feelings and communicate in a way that is focused on helping the other person rather than managing their own feelings.

It is important, therefore, as a nurse to respect any response that a person has to bad news or bereavement even if it is not the reaction that you personally would expect.

Grief and bereavement are different for individuals and the perception that a person needs to experience predetermined stages of grieving before they are regarded as 'over it' is perhaps not appropriate. For example, if a person cries when talking about a relative or friend that died one to two years previously, it may be perceived that they have not progressed through the bereavement stages and are having an abnormal bereavement reaction. Counselling is frequently seen as the solution to helping someone move on with their lives and sometimes individuals may find it useful. However Craib

(1999) believes that a different attitude towards grief and bereavement or death and dying can result in a very different approach to helping a person cope. 'Mourning never comes to an end; it is a process of remembering not one of leaving behind. The people we have lost live on within us and we can continue our relationship with them' (Craib 1999: 89).

By accepting that grief and bereavement is a normal reaction that can vary enormously between individuals rather than a series of stages to go through, a nurse can help a person deal with bad news or the death of a relative or friend in a more person-centred way. This means that by just being with the person and not having any expectations about how they should behave, the nurse may feel less anxious about how a person will react. The reaction of the person is almost irrelevant to how a nurse can help an individual or family, it is the reaction of the nurse that determines whether he/she can be supportive and helpful in this very difficult situation. The following actions by the nurse are important:

- Maintain a physical presence with the person or family – close physical presence or a discrete distance may be appropriate.
- Actively listen and let silence happen – this allows the person or family to think.
- Provide verbal and written information about what happens to the body and what the family need to do.

Supporting a person, or family, that has just lost a relative or friend is very emotionally draining and tiring for a nurse. When the bereaved have left the ward, the nurse might find it psychologically and physically helpful to take a break before getting on with the rest of the day's work.

One of the comments made frequently by students in relation to communication classes on dealing with grief and bereavement is that even if the class content is relevant, it still doesn't teach them how to do this in reality. This could be because students do not know what is expected from them in these situations when really, as we have seen from the above discussion, all that is required is an empathetic presence and the provision of information at the appropriate time regarding what happens next for the family. Other possible reasons why students and qualified staff nurses find it difficult to communicate include:

- Lack of confidence in relation to their own communication ability. Learning to be comfortable with silence and actively listen are the primary skills required when dealing with the dying and people who are bereaved.
- Dealing with death and dying at work on a regular basis can be a constant reminder of our own mortality and that of your family and friends. Spending time thinking about how you feel about death and your own spirituality could help you feel less anxious when helping others that are bereaved and grieving. Answering the exercise questions either on your own or with friends may help you identify your thoughts and feelings.

Exercise

How do you feel when you think about your own death?
Would you like to be cremated or buried when you die?
How would you like to die?
Do you believe in life after death?

Trying to answer these questions may make you feel uneasy but it will allow you to clearly separate your own personal views on death and dying from those of the people you care for at work. It means that when you communicate with people who are dying you are less fearful of questions like 'Nurse am I dying?' because, although the situation is still difficult, you may now be more comfortable with the emotions that you feel in relation to the topic, having explored them. This will allow you to give a patient-centred response, for example, 'What makes you think that you are dying'?

Cross-cultural communication

In the previous section we mentioned how people from different cultures often react to grief and bereavement in a very specific way. In this section the difficulties that can exist with communication between people from different cultural backgrounds because of the meaning attributed to various aspects of verbal and non-verbal communication will be discussed. Most societies are now multicultural and while this is not generally an issue of concern for people in their personal lives, it has considerable implications for those working in healthcare provision. The ability to provide intercultural care is based on an inherent respect for other people and a knowledge and understanding of the concept of culture and its influence on the behaviour of patients and nurses and other healthcare workers from different countries or those that represent different cultures within the same country.

Although often associated with race, the term 'ethnicity' actually refers to groups with a common cultural heritage and sense of identity. In contrast, the term 'race' is associated with biology, with members of a particular race sharing features such as skin colour (Giger and Davidhizar 1999). Ethnic and racial groups often overlap because of the biological and cultural similarities they share. Many definitions of culture exist but most share the common belief that culture represents the values, beliefs, norms and practices of a particular group that are learned, shared and guide thinking, decisions and actions in a specific way (Giger and Davidhizar 1999). Factors within ethnic groups, such as gender, age, education, religion, and socioeconomic status result in cultural diversity with an ethnic group. This means that for a nurse to care for patients with different cultural backgrounds in a patient-centred way they need to determine what aspects of a patient's culture are significant to their care and how this influences the way the nurse needs to communicate on an individual basis. Leininger (1991) refers to this process as 'transcultural nursing' and suggests that nurses need knowledge about many cultural values, beliefs and practices in order to provide individual and holistic nursing care. Nurses and midwives, however, do not always communicate well with patients with different cultural and religious backgrounds (Stockwell 1972; Jones and Van Amelsvoort-Jones 1986; Windsor-Richards and Gillies 1988, Wollett and Dosanjh-Matwala, 1990). This can be because if a nurse does not understand the patient's language they may avoid trying to communicate with the patient because it is embarrassing or time consuming. Waiting for the family to come in is a more efficient option. However, in the meantime the patient may be feeling isolated, uncomfortable and frightened. Often words are not necessary for a nurse to provide comfort and support when waiting for family or an interpreter to translate. Smiling or using gestures and gentle touch can be a very effective communication approach when trying to comfort and support a patient.

Some cultures are very expressive and use their hands, facial expression and voices to communicate in a way that can be perceived as argumentative or loud. This behaviour may also be perceived as unnecessary and aggressive by less-expressive cultures. A nurse may regard such behaviour as demanding or even aggressive and may avoid the patient or be defensive. The list of differences and similarities between cultures and ethnic groups is long and perhaps in terms of how a nurse communicates in a patient-centred way is irrelevant. We support Lea's (1994) view that for transcultural communication to be successful, nurses need to be aware of their own cultural values and attitudes and how these influence their perceptions of patients and the nursing care they give. This may sound familiar to you because we discuss the importance of developing awareness of how you communicate in order to be patient-centred in Chapters 3 and 9. The same principal applies for transcultural communication and helps prevent assumptions being made about a person's behaviour. In other words, the nurse can give a rational and non-judgmental response to patients regardless of their cultural or ethnic background.

Ethnocentrism may be a problem for nurses who are not aware of their own cultural values and attitudes. This is the perception that one's own way is best (Giger and Davidhizar 1999: 66). They suggest that nurses have a tendency towards ethnocentrism and this is evident in the way nurses often make assumptions about what patients need and provide nursing care without asking the patient what they want. For example, western culture views health and illness as a biophysical process and this is reflected in nurses' tendency to deal with the physical needs of a patient as separate from their psychological needs and well-being whereas other cultures such as some

Puerto Ricans believe that illness is related to evil while many Ugandans relate illness with being cursed (Grypma 1993). Awareness of oneself as a unique individual with a cultural and ethnic background allows a nurse to view others also as unique individuals with individual needs and provide patient-centred care. Methods of developing self-awareness will be further developed in Chapter 9.

Key points

▶ Situations are sometimes perceived as 'difficult' by nurses because of a perceived lack of communication skills.

▶ Ordinary everyday situations can become 'difficult' because nurses' communicate inappropriately or negatively.

▶ Observing a 'good' role model is a very effective way of developing effective and positive communication skills.

▶ The key to managing 'difficult' situations is to learn to 'manage you'. This requires self-awareness, motivation and practice.

▶ A key role of the nurse in situations relating to death/dying, bereavement and bad news is to provide comfort and information that is helpful, relevant and patient-centred.

▶ Learning to managing anxiety (nurses and patients) will alleviate, or possibly prevent, many 'difficult' situations.

▶ Awareness of personal cultural values and attitudes is essential in preventing ethnocentrism and allows nurses to care for patients from other cultures in a patient-centred and individualized way.

PART III

The Development of Therapeutic Communication Skills

9 Values and Beliefs in Nursing

Introduction

The purpose of this chapter is to explore the values, beliefs and attitudes inherent in the nursing profession and how these influence communication and nursing practice. Students will find this chapter useful because it provides an explanation about what makes the work of a nurse unique within health-care professions and how the values and beliefs that nurses hold about nursing are evident in how they communicate with patients, families and work colleagues. Concepts such as personal and professional values, ethics in nursing, professionalism and accountability will be discussed under separate headings. However, it is important to note that these concepts are inextricably linked in how they influence the practice and development of nursing.

Values

Values are made up of the beliefs and attitudes a person holds about everything in life. The values a person holds gives them meaning in what they do, how they appreciate their environment and people and guide how they react to situations in life (Rich 2007; Tschudin 2003). Values change and develop as we experience various aspects of life and often we are not aware of our values until they are tested, for example, a nurse may discover that although she does not agree with a patient refusing to undergo chemotherapy for the treatment of cancer, they value human rights and the patient's right to choose their treatment. The nurse, therefore, accepts the patient's decision and cares for them in this context.

Beliefs are influenced and guided by values, for example, a nurse may hold the value that every human being is a unique individual. In nursing this belief will translate into the belief that maintaining the dignity and respect of a patient is the primary function of the nurse and should be reflected in the care that is given by the nurse.

An attitude is evident in a person's disposition and is formed by their values and beliefs. This can have a positive or negative influence on how a person communicates. Most of us recognize a positive or negative attitude in the way a person communicates verbally and non-verbally. In nursing, the belief that patients should do as they are told because the doctor/ nurse knows best will translate into an attitude whereby the nurse does not respect the right of the individual to choose their treatment or even be involved in decisions about their treatment. This nurse may argue with the patient, try to coerce them and generally disregard the patient's viewpoint. This type of communication is not patient centred and the patient may even be labelled as 'difficult'. The attitude or disposition of a nurse is influenced by their upbringing and environment but also and probably most importantly the values and beliefs they hold about human beings and the role of the nurse.

 Exercise

What values to you hold about nursing and your role as a nurse? If you are not sure, ask yourself the following questions:

Why did I choose nursing as a career?
What aspects of my job do I like the most?
What aspects of my job do I like the least?

Be honest with yourself when considering the answers to these questions, otherwise the exercise will not help you identify your real values about nursing and the role of the nurse. Knowing what you value about your job will give meaning to the job you do and may even boost your self-esteem. However, consider the answers carefully because as you read on you will see that your values impact greatly on how you do your job!

Defining nursing is generally regarded as problematic as the work is often regarded as invisible. This poses difficulties for nurses in communicating accurately with other healthcare professionals about what nursing is (Rutherford 2008; Bowker et al. 2001). The effect of this is that nurses may not feel they control nursing, influence practice by putting nursing into public policy or defend/argue for nursing's financing (Clark and Lang 1992). There have been many attempts to define nursing, for example, Virginia Henderson (1966) described the function of the nurse as 'assist the individual, sick or well, in the performance of those activities contributing to health or its recovery (or to a peaceful death) that he would perform unaided if he had the necessary strength, will or knowledge. And to do this in such a way as to help him gain independence as rapidly as possible'.

This definition is useful in providing a broad view of what nursing aspires to but further consideration suggests that this definition could also apply to other healthcare disciplines such as physiotherapists, occupational therapists and doctors and does not give a sense of the complexity of the collaborative and interdisciplinary communication and working required to provide high-quality patient-centred care. Also, what is lacking in this definition is the recognition of the integral contribution that the values, beliefs and attitudes of individual nurses make to the implementation of this role. In other words, how the nurse communicates this role to the patient (McCabe and Timmins 2012).

In earlier chapters we discussed Rogers (1961) person-centred theory and how the personal characteristics of warmth, genuineness and unconditional positive regard are required to be person-centred. These characteristics go hand-in hand with the personal values that regard human beings as unique individuals that deserve to be treated with respect and dignity. A person-centred attitude or approach to patient care will be evident in nurses with these values and characteristics. However, if a nurse does not have these characteristics or does not value patients as unique individuals, then it is likely that their attitude or approach to patient care is task-centred.

Rutty (1998: 249) put forward another view that 'nurses are managers of health who coordinate and care for patients/clients health throughout their life continuum, both within the acute sector and the community. … it is the nurse who "knows" the patient and utilizes all the other healthcare professionals and disciplines in organizing that care'. This is an interesting definition of the role of the nurse because is more specific than Henderson's (1966) and acknowledges that caring for patients is an interdisciplinary process. In using the term 'utilizes' to describe the working relationship between nurses and other healthcare professionals Rutty (1998) also implied that nurses were superior to all other health professionals and have other disciplines' knowledge and skills at their disposal. By substituting the term 'utilizes' with 'works collaboratively with' Rutty's (1998) definition goes a long way towards defining nursing in a modern context, while at the same time revealing the uniqueness of the nursing role in caring for patients within the healthcare system. Nurses 'know' the patient better than any other healthcare worker because they spend time with them and they see the physiotherapists, doctors and occupational therapists come and go. The nurse coordinates the contribution of other healthcare professions to patient care in a way that is therapeutic and patient-centred.

Nurses' coordinate and provide patient/client care in many different contexts including acute/chronic and community settings. The nurse interprets and translates information for the patient and helps the patient and family derive meaning from the information they receive from other healthcare disciplines. The nurse communicates between disciplines and across disciplines about patient care and specific patient needs. The nurse does this effectively and successfully because she 'knows' the patient as a person and a patient.

Reed (2011) provides a more contemporary and comprehensive view of what nursing is, which reflects many of these aspects of nursing. She describes it as a way of working and being with people that facilitates well-being. Nursing creates knowledge and practice based on complexity and integration that is experienced as well-being in people that nurses care for. This description of nursing acknowledges the many facets of nursing in meeting its ultimate goal of facilitating well-being in others. The level of personal self-awareness and communication competence required by each individual nurse to achieve this is significant.

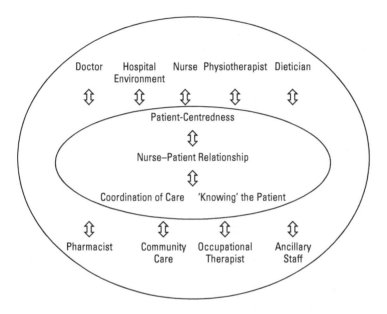

Figure 9.1   A model of nursing within the context of collaborative and patient-centred care

Figure 9.1 represents a model of nursing within the context of collaborative and patient-centred care.

This model illustrates the context of the nurse–patient relationship in relation to all the other healthcare disciplines and services. The double arrow indicates that communication between the nurse and patient is two way and collaborative.

Advocacy

Advocacy exists in many forms including legal advocacy, self-advocacy, collective advocacy and citizen advocacy (Bateman 2000; Gates 1994). A legal advocate is a person who is legally trained and works within legislative frameworks in representing the rights and interests of others. A self-advocate is a person who encourages and helps others in developing confidence and self-esteem. Collective advocacy is when an organization supports a specific group of people. For example, Amnesty International exclusively supports those whose human rights have been violated. Citizen advocacy is probably best known for the support of those with physical and intellectual disabilities. When the parents or guardian of a person with disabilities dies the state appoints a person who can work with that person in meeting their needs.

Advocacy promotes and defends the individualism of patients and is based on an ethical construct and is an integral role of all healthcare professionals (McDonald 2007; Llewellyn 2004). Although not exclusive to nursing, advocacy is a concept often referred to as an integral role of nursing (Hanks 2010; Negarandeh 2006).

An advocate is 'a person who publicly supports or recommends a particular cause or policy or makes a case on someone else's behalf' (*Oxford English Dictionary* 2012). In nursing advocacy is every nurse's professional duty and is grounded in patients' legal and moral rights (Vaartio et al. 2008). A nurse becomes an advocate by being responsible for meeting the patients' needs and through nursing activities carried out for the patient and family. The rights referred to in this description of an advocate include:

- A right or healthcare.
- A right to a reasonable standard of care.
- A right to give consent.
- A right of access to health records.
- A right to confidentiality.
- A right to complain. (Dimond 1999)

Increased awareness of their rights means that patients now exercise their rights in questioning doctors and nurses about their treatment and care, making choices about where they get treatment and who gives it and having access to all information relating to their care. Nurses advocate for patients in many ways but perhaps primarily in everyday activities by helping patients make choices that meet their needs, for example, how to get out of bed safely, what is the most appropriate food (Llewellyn, 2004). However, there are issues for nurses in limiting their ability of carry out the advocacy role. These include the lack of power that nurses have in the context of healthcare provision. This means that rather than advocating for patients as a group at local or national level, for example, in implanting health promotion strategies, nurses are limited to advocating for patients on an individual basis. This too is limited because advocating for a patient can have negative impact on the nurse. Doctors and other healthcare disciplines may not like nurses 'interfering' in decisions about patient care and being a successful advocate requires communication skills such as assertiveness and negotiation. Without these skills, nurses often resort to very covert actions when advocating for patients particularly in situations where the various healthcare disciplines do not work collaboratively.

Example

A nurse accompanies a doctor who tells an elderly patient that he has cancer of the stomach but that the doctors will remove it in an operation. The doctor says that she will return later with the consent form for the patient to sign. The nurse was concerned that the patient had not received enough detail about the surgery or how it would affect the patients' quality of life. So when the doctor had gone, the nurse asked the patient if they understood everything the doctor said. The patient said no and wondered how he would feel after the surgery. The nurse told him that he would have most of his stomach removed in a surgical procedure that would require the patient to spend time in intensive care and he would only be able to eat small amounts of liquidized food in future. Immediately the patient said to the nurse 'I don't want that, I am 78 years old and I like my food. I'd rather continue on the way I am for as long as I can'. The nurse reassured the patient that if that were his decision then he would not have to have surgery. The doctor was very irate when the patient told her he would not give consent for surgery and confronted the nurse who explained that when given the facts, it was the patient's right to decide how they wanted to spend the rest of his life.

This example gives an indication of how the boundaries between advocacy and ethical issues can be blurred and also indicates why the development and use of assertiveness skills is so important in nursing. It would be very difficult and very frustrating for a nurse to advocate for a patient if they cannot use assertive skills.

Example
A patient has a respiratory arrest on a ward. The 'arrest team' come to the ward and as they begin resuscitation the senior doctor asks the age of the patient. The nurse replies 89. The whole team seem to hesitate and consider whether this is in the best interests of the patient but the nurse quickly points out that this patient is fully ambulatory, independent and due for discharge the following day. The team continues resuscitation that is successful and the patient is discharged a few days later.

This is an example of how knowing the patient and valuing the person as an individual influences the advocacy role.

Ethics in nursing

The word 'ethics' is a Greek word that means character and is concerned with systems and behaviour that guide right and wrong. Systems that are ethical are accountable and transparent but do not dictate individual human behaviour. Ethics does not provide definitive guidelines for behaviour. Ethical principles related to truth, goodness, justice and freedom form a framework within which ethical issues can be considered. It is the values we hold as human beings that influences the way we live and conduct our lives morally and ethically. This is true also of our role as nurses. Values we hold as nurses and about nursing influence the way we communicate with people and make moral and ethical decisions about their care. Listening, a core communication that was discussed in Chapter 4 lies at the heart of ethics and being ethical requires commitment, responsibility, attention, reasoning and intelligence (Tschudin 2003). These characteristics and skills are necessary for one to be ethical but also for one to be a nurse that is patient-centred and therapeutic. This takes place within the context of 'knowing the patient' and the uniqueness of nursing within healthcare practices. This may also be the reason why nurses and doctors can sometimes disagree about patient care. Nursing ethics sometimes conflict with that of other professions because the importance of developing and sustaining a nurse–patient relationship is a fundamental nursing value. Other professions may not understand this because communication between physiotherapists and patients, for example, is focused on mobility or breathing exercises and is usually transient.

Gaudine et al. (2011) report that ethical conflict, for doctors and nurses, arises from key areas, for example:

- disagreement about care decisions or treatment options;
- others not respecting a patient's wishes;
- patient not receiving quality end-of-life care;
- patient's or family's behaviour preventing safe or quality care for self or others;
- patient and/or family not having informed consent or full disclosure;
- not knowing the 'right thing to do';
- system deficit or deficiency preventing quality care;
- nurse or physician values conflict with patient values or lifestyle choices; and
- possible or perceived deficiencies in care owing to nurse or physician competency.

Example
An 82 year old lady named Elizabeth had an extensive cerebrovascular accident four days ago and is unresponsive. The doctor has said that she should have a PEG tube inserted. The nurse who has been caring for this patient and her family is concerned that this course of treatment is not what the patient or her family would want. Over the previous 4 days the family had talked about the patient with the nurse. They told her what

the lady used to look like, how she liked to dress up and wear her pearls every day and play cards with her friends every Saturday night. She was a great golfer and kept a perfect garden. They expressed enormous sorrow that she would not be able to do these things again and felt that she would not like to live without her independence and quality of life. When the nurse expressed her view that a PEG tube may not be the most appropriate course of treatment for this patient, the doctor was dismissive and said there was not another option. The nurse persisted and suggested that the doctor discuss the issue with the family. The doctor said it had already been discussed with the family who had given their consent. The nurse felt that the family did not fully understand the implications of this course of treatment and talked to the nurse manager. The nurse manager did not agree with the nurse and indicated that she did not wish to continue discussing the matter. The nurse was upset by this and felt that she could not influence the situation.

This is an example of what can happen in reality when nurses consider a particular course of treatment as ethically wrong. The nurse felt that the treatment was futile and served only to prolong the patient's suffering and that as a result of coming to 'know her patient' through the family, this is not what the patient would have wanted. The difference in viewpoint comes from the different values they hold as doctor and nurse and the way in which both professions interpret the ethical aspects of patient care. The outcome of the above interaction is not a positive one and the nurse is left feeling 'let down' by her manager. But this is an example of where there is no right or wrong answer. The doctor, nurse and nurse manager could all justify their views and actions professionally and ethically. Junior nurses can find a situation like this particularly difficult and often when faced with the opinions of senior nurses that are based on a different set of personal and professional values, they tend to avoid the situation or remain passive. However, this can also occur in experienced nurses especially if they perceive that they are unsupported by their manager. The outcome of this avoidance and passive behaviour is a feeling of powerlessness and inferiority (Peter et al. 2004).

Exercise

How could the nurse have dealt differently with the situation? What would you have done?

When confronted with opposing views it is important to use assertive behaviour that is confrontational. This is an essential communication skill for nurses to acquire in their professional development. Chapter 7 outlines how to be assertive. Remember, being ethical also requires commitment, reasoning and intelligence and this in conjunction with assertive skills means that you do not feel powerless or inferior. Instead you feel that as a nurse and because you 'know the patient' you are ethically bound to verbalize your concerns regarding their treatment. This type of communication is integral to the development of interdisciplinary collaborative relationships in caring for patients. Working collaboratively does not mean that each discipline, for example, nurses, doctors, physiotherapists, do not have their own agendas. They do but, the patient is at the core of their actions and it is the way in which each member of the healthcare team communicates and does their work that indicates whether it is ethical and moral or not (Liaschenko and Peter 2004). The nurse in the scenario above could have persisted even though it would have been difficult for her given the view of her manager and the doctors. By discussing the situation further with the family and establishing whether or not they understood the implications for the patient of inserting a PEG tube, the nurse may have been able to identify issues that needed further discussion. On this basis, dialogue between the doctor and family would need to continue before the tube was inserted with the nurse being more vocal about what was best for the patient as a unique individual.

Nursing as a profession

The key elements of a profession include factors such as autonomy, monopoly, expertise, integrity, service and rewards (Basford and Slevin 2003). Nursing has worked hard over the past century to become and be recognized as a profession. This encompasses characteristics such as a unique body of knowledge, code of ethics, control over work and autonomy in practice to name a few. However, not all agree that nursing can or should be a profession because nursing is rooted in practice and by pursuing academic qualifications nurses would not be as caring towards their patients. Nurses appear to disagree with this view and perceive themselves as intelligent, self-governing and professional especially since the development of specialist and advanced nursing roles (Shaw and Degazon 2008; Takase et al. 2001). Traditionally, professions claim to hold ethical values that are demonstrated in codes of professional conduct and have given professions the power to act without reference to external agencies (Colyer 2004). This level of autonomy was previously the exclusive right of groups such as doctors and lawyers. However, with the development of patients' charters and legislation such as the Freedom of Information Act even these groups are required to more transparent in their accountability. Furthermore, given the consistently fluctuating demands on healthcare services and the external forces that influence the structure and organization of healthcare it is difficult for all healthcare professions to control their work and environment. This means that perhaps autonomy at such a level is no longer realistic especially within the healthcare context. With the development of numerous professional bodies within healthcare such as physiotherapy, therapeutic radiography and occupational therapy, medicine is no longer the dominant profession. The question is perhaps not related to whether nursing is a profession or not but rather whether it is equal to others in a healthcare context. Colyer (2004) suggests that nursing is not equal to other professions, not because nurses do not believe nursing to be equal and that is an important attribute for any profession but because of the distorted and stereotypical image of nurses and nursing that is held by the public as a result of media influences. Hart (2004) suggests that image is not that important and the experience of people as patients or consumers is more influential in how nurses are perceived

The strength of nursing as a profession lies in its ethical basis that values the uniqueness of individuals and patient autonomy above other healthcare professionals (Redman and Fry 2000). For nurses to be recognized as equal by the public within the interdisciplinary delivery of healthcare they need to communicate as equals. This means communicating assertively, developing negotiating skills and communicate collectively by supporting, respecting and encouraging each other. As discussed in Chapter 7, working collaboratively with other disciplines requires these skills. Becoming equal members of the interdisciplinary healthcare team not just in the delivery of healthcare at the bedside but also at local and national level in the development and implementation of healthcare policy and resource allocation requires political behaviour and motivation. As any successful politician knows, effective and positive interpersonal communication is essential in gaining the respect of others. Nurses need to be political and recognize the fundamental importance of positive and effective communication so that they will be instigators of healthcare reform and successful change agents rather than having change done to them. It is important to remember this will occur within an interdisciplinary context and nurses should be mindful and respectful of other disciplines. For change initiatives and healthcare services to be patient focused this process must be collaborative and although disciplines will still have their own agenda and compete for resources, the focus for all negotiation and communication should be the provision of a patient-centred high-quality interdisciplinary care service. Nurses and nursing are best placed to maintain a patient-centred focus.

Nursing has been described as an art and a science with art representing the unique skilful practice of nursing and science representing knowledge and the provision of evidence to support practice. Nurse theorists and educators have discussed and debated this issue for many years as a means of identifying key elements of nursing that are unique to nursing. Like all healthcare professions nurses are trying to distinguish themselves from other disciplines especially medicine and in doing so attain status and power. Perhaps nursing needs to consider whether this is necessary or appropriate in becoming a profession and recognize that nursing and medicine are interdependent as are all other healthcare disciplines when providing care for patients. Conflict is probably inevitable but, as you will have read in Chapter 6, conflict is not the problem: the problem is how to respond to it or manage it successfully. Collaborative communication is the key to managing conflict successfully and is also the key to placing nursing within the interdisciplinary healthcare team on an equal but distinct footing with other disciplines. Leaders from nursing and medicine should lead the way in developing collaborative working environments. However, there is an individual responsibility to communicate collaboratively. This is not just from a nursing perspective as all healthcare disciplines need to communicate collaboratively but for nursing collaborative communication will have a positive impact on the way nursing is viewed by other healthcare disciplines and as nurses become more political and regarded as equal in terms of healthcare professions the public may also change their stereotypical view of nursing.

Accountability

Accountability is referred to as 'an important legal, ethical, and moral term reflecting an attitude of human obligation to other persons, groups, organizations, and societies' (Milton 2008: 300). The term accountability has been used in nursing as a means of strengthening its status as a profession and is generally included in professional scope and standards of nursing practice or code of ethical conduct documents. Individual nurses are accountable for their clinical decision making and nursing care provided. In day-to-day terms this means that nurses must always be prepared and able to explain and justify their professional practice to relevant stakeholders (Milton 2008).

Hancock (1997) argued that nurses do not have the authority to act in a way that they think is best for the patient, therefore, cannot be truly accountable. Mason (2011) reports that nurses are still excluded from policy-making processes and while such current power structures exists in healthcare provision at local, national and international level nursing has a significant challenge to be truly accountable. Chapter 7 has addressed the issues in relation to the communication skills required to credibly and effectively contribute to health and healthcare policy development. This is an important point not just in relation to accountability but also professionalism, advocacy and autonomy in nursing.

Clinical governance provides a framework that could be very useful in bringing about the changes needed to develop a high-quality and patient-centred healthcare service. This is a framework where healthcare staff are collectively accountable for the quality of patient care (McSherry and Pearce 2011). Healthcare managers and the numerous healthcare professions work together on the understanding of mutual trust and respect of all involved. This framework embraces and encourages experiential and collaborative learning and development within and between healthcare professions. The implications of the clinical governance framework for nursing are twofold. The first benefit to nursing is that authority and equality will exist within the context of providing high-quality, patient-centred care. The second benefit for nursing and other healthcare professions is that the power associated with, and claimed by, medicine will be diluted. Clearly, therefore, the introduction of clinical governance is not be easy and while on paper it seems idealistic to think such a framework can bring about such a radical cultural and organizational change in attitude, the fact that it exists and is proposed at governmental level is most significant.

The underlying emphasis on individual responsibility and accountability in the delivery of high-quality care and self/professional regulation is perhaps the most significant part of this framework. This recognizes how our personal and professional values regarding the role of the nurse, nursing as a profession and the patient influence our practice and that without this individual commitment to open, collaborative communication that has the patients needs at its core, very little will change!

Key points

▶ The values, beliefs and attitudes that a nurse holds about nursing, patients and people generally are reflected in the way they communicate and care for patients.

▶ A nurse's awareness of his/her values helps them identify if the way they communicate is patient-centred or task-centred.

▶ The 'uniqueness' of nursing within healthcare provision lies in 'knowing the patient' and coordinating interdisciplinary care. This role needs to be valued and protected by nurses with the context of healthcare development and planning at national and local level.

▶ Collaborative care is essential in providing care that is holistic and patient-centred. Nurses need to embrace this and actively pursue it using political nursing leadership.

▶ In order to be professional, nurses need to be ethical, patient advocates, accountable and autonomous. To do this nurses need to value the work they do as equal members of a collaborative interdisciplinary healthcare team. An essential communication skill in achieving this is assertive behaviour.

10 The Role of Self-Awareness in Developing Therapeutic Communication Skills

Introduction

We have spent some time in previous chapters discussing elements of the therapeutic relationship that nurses can build with patients in their care. According to Arnold and Underman Boggs (2011) self-awareness is essential for successful implementation of this therapeutic relationship, and something that services users believe to be of great importance (Department of Health 2012). Other authors go so far as to say that not being aware of self can lead to communication problems in the nurse–patient relationship (Betts 2003) or interfere with the smooth running of this relationship (Kantcheva and Eckroth-Bucher 2002). This chapter considers the meaning of self-awareness in the context of contemporary healthcare and outlines ways to develop and improve self-awareness.

Developing awareness

Before discussing self-awareness it is worth spending time considering what we mean by self-awareness. Kantcheva and Eckroth-Bucher (2002) suggest that understanding of others begins with understanding oneself. They also suggest that a lack of self-awareness, or self-understanding, can interfere with the nurse–client relationship. For example, past experiences, attitudes, and responses to specific client populations or circumstances can affect the behaviour of the nurse. Therefore negative reactions, biases, prejudices and stereotyping must be recognized and explored through self-awareness.

Exercise

Write out reasons why you think self-awareness may be important in nursing. Write two to three lines.

You may have mentioned some or all of the following as suggested reasons for the development of self-awareness in nurses:

- to enhance self-understanding,
- to allow acceptance of others,
- to become equipped with dealing with difficult situations,
- to enable self-monitoring, and
- to enhance personal autonomy. (Burnard 1997)

This list shows how useful self-awareness can be in many nursing situations.

What is self-awareness?

Perhaps no aspect of mind is more familiar or more puzzling than consciousness and our conscious experience of self and world. (Stanford Encyclopedia of Philosophy, 2012)

Indeed Seager (2012) suggests that we as humans are not good at self-understanding.

Exercise

What does self-awareness mean to you? Write two to three lines.

Self-awareness is a broad overarching concept that includes our physical awareness of our bodies, our sense of being spatially situated, our social situatedness (awareness of reactions to others in social situations) and introspection (ability to examine one's thoughts and motivations (Seager 2012). The *Oxford English Dictionary* (2012) defined self-awareness as 'conscious knowledge of one's own character, feelings, motives and desires'. Interestingly an additional note with this citation is 'the process can be painful but it leads to greater self-awareness' (Oxford English Dictionary 2012) indicating perhaps the modern approach to enhancing and developing this aspect of self.

Burnard (1985: 15) describes self-awareness as a 'gradual and continuous process of noticing and exploring aspects of self, whether behavioural, psychological or physical with the intention of developing personal and interpersonal understanding'. While consensus regarding a definition is not evident, self-awareness is an espoused virtue in nursing and refers to the nurse being aware of their verbal and non-verbal behaviours and intentions and how this impacts the therapeutic relationship.

Exercise

Karen a staff nurse that you are working with has a tendency to frown.
Can you think what message this frown may send to patients unintentionally?
Can you identify ways that Karen could become aware of this habit?

You may have suggested that the client may interpret this frowning in a negative way, perhaps sensing anger or frustration from the nurse. You may have suggested that a peer review of Karen's role may reveal this tendency to frown or you may have suggested reflection. Reflection is gaining increasing popularity within the nursing profession. Indeed, it is espoused that nurses become reflective practitioners. Methods such as this for increasing self-awareness will be considered later in the chapter. However, the meaning of 'self' and 'self-awareness' require some discussion in the interim.

Burnard's (1997) Model of Self

- The physical aspect of self
- The real self
- The ideal self
- The self-for-others
- The social self
- The spiritual self
- The darker aspect of self
- The sexual self

Figure 10.1 Burnard's Model of Self

Source: adapted from Burnard, P. (1997) *Know Yourself! Self-Awareness Activities for Nurses and Other Health Professionals*, London: Whurr Publishers Limited.

Awareness

Awareness is often described as a human feature. Unlike animals, humans, through consciousness, are aware of themselves, their thoughts, feelings, behaviour and physical and emotional self. Self-awareness the ability to perceive one's own existence, including feelings and behaviours, it is a personal understanding of one's identity. At a basic level, each human has an awareness of self. There is a consciousness and awareness of those aspects of self as described in Figure 10.1.

However, within nursing self-awareness has become associated with a developmental process of getting to know the self more. A key author in this area, Burnard (1985, 1997) highlights the increased development of self-awareness as a positive element in nurses and a requirement of professional nursing practice. Through developing a greater awareness of self, elements of self can be explored and developed in order to improve communication skills (Burnard 1997).

Self

There is a significant body of psychological literature that examines the concept of self. There are multiple complex notions interpretations and understandings of self, awareness and consciousness (Stanford Encyclopedia of Philosophy 2012). However, for the purposes of this book we are aiming to develop a basic understanding of self, in order to build a specific self-awareness in communications that will improve your nursing practice in this area. DeVito (2011: 26) describes the notion of 'self-concept' as your notion of who you think you are.

Psychological theorists who explore the nature of self and are commonly associated with communication in nursing include Sigmund Freud and Carl Rogers (1961) (Chapter 3). Freud proposed the notion of the unconscious self whereby individual's reactions in situations may be unconscious and linked to past experiences such as those in childhood. A number of unconscious defence mechanisms are also outlined, such as denial, repression, displacement and reaction formation. Self-awareness is not referred to explicitly within this theory. As self-awareness requires self-consciousness, the unconscious nature of individuals as proposed by Freud, with complex ego defence mechanisms warrant self-exploration a difficult and highly specialized task, possibly requiring professional assistance.

Behaviourism on the other hand oversimplifies the human condition, reducing it to one of response to stimulus to the external environment. Human self-awareness and self-consciousness is restricted as they are reactors rather than being in control of their own behaviours (Ellis et al. 2003).

The humanistic model pays greater attention to self-awareness. Rogers (1961) asserted that humans are dynamic reactive individuals who seek to achieve their full potential. Humans are motivated towards continual self-improvement.

Peplau (1991) described how the self develops from appraisals made by self and significant others about self, as an infant and child. Continued repetition of these appraisals becomes a pattern that is incorporated into self. With each new era of development, the self may be reappraised. Thus, Peplau (1991) asserts that the development of self is an ongoing process that continues throughout life.

Burnard (1997) provided a simple model of self. Using this model the self may be conceptualized as containing multiple and interrelated aspects of self that come together to form a whole (see Figure 10.1). Burnard (1997: 7) describes the physical self as the '*bodily* sense of self' (emphasis added). He suggested that communication occurs 'through our physical sense of self' that is through non-verbal communication, which he described as 'body language' (1997: 7). Body language includes eye contact, touch, gesture, proximity to others, non-verbal aspects of speech and facial expression.

Exercise

Sit quietly for a moment. Become aware of your body. Take 10 deep breaths in and out, close your eyes and consider what parts of your body you are aware of. Write two to three lines on this experience.

You might notice from doing this exercise that you became aware of your arms, your hand, your legs and your feet, and perhaps some other parts of your body. Did you notice that you became more conscious of these then you would be normally? Usually in our act of being consciously aware we don't register all the body parts all of the time. This is an automatic component of being aware that we sometimes take for granted. However, using this exercise to become aware of your body may be useful in becoming aware of your reactions. If you become aware of your body in a communication setting you might notice that your fists are clenched. Realizing that this could be perceived as anger to others (or indeed increase your anger) (see Chapter 8) you may (having become aware) unclench them. This is an example of how self-awareness (in one area) can improve your communication skills.

Communication models for increasing self-awareness

A move away from ritualistic and task based nursing is required to encourage nurses away from the use of linear models of communication. These latter focus on the basic principles of communication (message-sender-receiver) and although the message may be communicated, there is little consideration of the relationship. Chapter 3 also identified partnership as an important theme in the contemporary use of conceptual models of nursing (Pearson et al. 2005). The development of the nurse/patient relationship was identified as crucial to this process (Orem 2001). When non-linear models of communication are used the therapeutic relationship becomes increasingly important (Comforting Interaction-Relationship Model- Morse et al. 1997).

There is an unconscious nature to all communication interactions, as referred to in Chapter 3, which suggests a certain unawareness of our personal contribution to some interactions. For example, relatives in O'Shea's (2004) study found that recognition and a wave from nurses [that had previously nursed their infant] held significant value for them in the hospital environment, a fact of which these nurses may be totally unaware. Similarly, words and body language that nurses chose to use when approaching patients affected the extent to which communication was patient-centred. Timmins et al. (2005) highlight that small behaviours have potentially great impact across a variety of nursing situations, and suggested that small gestures can make a difference. Griffits (Timmins et al 2005) termed these 'microbehaviours', which have increased significance in situations where individuals have cognitive dysfunction.

However, the challenge remains for nurses to examine these microbehaviours to ascertain their impact on the development of the therapeutic relationship with patients. While nurse communication texts have typically drawn on psychological theories that explain and predict behaviour, preferred models for the development of self-awareness have traditionally been a rather simplified version of these. Burnard (1997) for example suggested the use of the Johari Window, originally developed by Luft (1984) (Figure 10.2).

In this model different aspects of a person are represented in each of the four window areas. DeVito (2011: 27) refers to this as 'the four selves'. The 'open' quadrant represents things that you know about yourself that others also know. The 'blind' quadrant represents things that others may know about you, but which you are unaware of. The 'hidden' quadrant

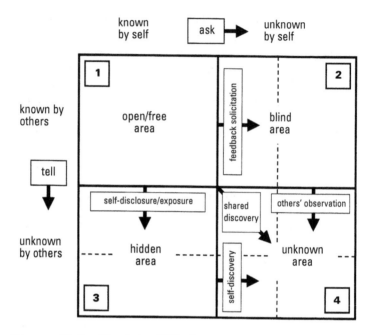

Figure 10.2   The Johari Window

Source: Luft, J. (1984) *Group Process: an Introduction to Group Dynamics (3rd ed)* New York : McGraw Hill. Reproduced with permission from The McGraw-Hill Companies, Inc

represents things that you know about yourself that others do not. The 'unknown' quadrant represents things that neither you nor others know about you. This model allows for use of psychological theories as mentioned earlier. The unknown quadrant could refer to Freud's unconscious reactions or defence mechanisms, or to behaviourist responses to the environment.

Rogers (1961) suggested that some degree of self-disclosure benefits relationships and increases self-esteem. However, psychology is a highly specialized field and in some cases an analysis of self may require professional assistance. Although it has been suggested that use of the Johari Window use requires a 'trained, experienced facilitator' (Rowe 1999), and certainly it may be useful in this context, writers have largely suggested that professional assistance is not required, and have suggested that it is something that you can use yourself to develop a greater self-awareness (De Vito 2011; Burnard 1997).

The basic concept of the Johari Window allows us to examine our hidden selves through disclosure and feedback from others. These processes of disclosure and feedback can enhance the sense of self, and promote self-awareness, in a way similar to Burnard (1997). Burnard (1997: 9) described the real self as one that is personal and not usually known by a wide circle of acquaintances. It is essentially private and described as 'internal'. Burnard (1997) suggested that items in the hidden dimension are common to many people and are not disclosed. Burnard (1997: 10) also argued that perhaps there is no real self, but that we play out a series of roles in our lives. Our real self is little more than a 'collection of scripts and roles that we acquire over the years of our life'.

There is also the notion of ideal self, which Burnard suggested is the 'day dream about how we would like to be' (1997: 11). This may originate from ideas that we have about how others live their lives. The ideal self is therefore a 'picture in our heads' (1997: 11). The self for others is those aspects of self that we present and is dependent on our relationship with them. The social self relates to how we present ourselves in groups. For Burnard the spiritual self is described as 'often associated with religion, (but) it need not necessarily be so' (1997: 15). It is equated by Burnard (1997) with individuals seeking meaning and purpose in their lives. Burnard (1997) contends that this is another very personal aspect of the self that sometimes people do not wish to discuss.

The hidden self, Burnard (1997) suggests, relates to the 'skeletons in the cupboard' (1997: 19). These may be aspects of the self that 'we do not particularly like' (1997: 19). These include: aggressive feelings towards others, sexual thoughts and feelings, and thoughts and feelings that we perceive to be unusual to ourselves and not necessarily shared by others. With regard to the sexual self, Burnard (1997) described two distinct aspects: sexual orientation and sexual identity. The latter refers to whether an individual is male or female and the former refers to the sexual orientation. Expression of sexuality within sexual orientation can occur in many ways including:

heterosexual orientation (expression of sexual attraction to persons of the opposite sex); homosexual (expression of sexual attraction to persons of the same sex); and bisexual (expression of sexual attraction to persons of the both the same and opposite sex) (Burnard 1977). From all of this you can see that knowing yourself is a complex task.

Exercise

Using the Johari Window complete each of the following sections:

Open self: write two to three lines about yourself that others know.

Hidden self: write two to three lines about your hidden self that others don't know.

Pause to consider these.

Now see if you can consider:

Blind self: what you think others know about you that you don't know.

Unknown self: can you think of anything unknown about yourself?

Now using the Johari Window ask a friend or family member to complete the four quadrants using information about you.

Take time to compare the two versions and see if you can add any information to your blind self and unknown self quadrants.

Tip: focus this exercise on you as a nurse if you would like this exercise focused.

Hopefully from this exercise you will have discovered things about yourself that you were not fully aware of, thus showing how the blind self and unknown self can be present. At the same time you will probably realize that increasing your knowledge of these elements can help you to develop by either increasing your confidence or making you realize that you have things that you need to work on and improve.

Other methods to promote self-awareness include beginning to understand and read one's own emotions and recognize their impact. DeVito (2011: 28) suggests that the following are necessary steps to grow in self-awareness:

- listening to what others have to say about you,
- increase your open self,
- seek information about yourself, and
- dialogue with yourself ('no one knows you better than yourself').

Through self-awareness and recognition of emotions valuable information can be learned. You can build personal strength from acknowledging your 'weakness'. Good methods of developing self-awareness include asking others for feedback, engaging a critical friend to review your strengths and weaknesses and taking personality tests (such as those found on Queendom.com (2012). While you may not have access to professional assistance for your exercise above, it is important when you choose someone to assist you with your self-development that you choose someone with relevant knowledge and skills or life experience and also someone that you can trust. You might like to call this person a critical friend. This is someone that you can trust to disclose your intimate feelings with and with whom you will feel safe. You are looking for someone that is trustworthy, approachable, reliable, a good listener, flexible, supportive, consistent and open, and willing to share a little of themselves. Check through this list of characteristics to find someone suitable. Disclosure to develop self-awareness usually takes place in a 'dyad' (two people) rather than in a group, and predominately occurs in a situation where there is honest mutual disclosure (De Vito 2011). This does not mean that this critical friend/ mentor needs to be overly personal, however, in the clinical area they may be able to identify particular episodes from their own student experience that may help you.

Another suggestion is to develop a list of situations at work that sparked emotional reactions or were difficult to resolve. Write a few sentences for each situation describing what happened, how you felt, what you said, what the other person said, how it turned out. Through this writing themes and possible triggers can be identified to help modify reactions in similar situations in the future. Other suggestions included setting aside half an hour daily for reflection and/or keeping a journal to record insights, feelings and daily situations.

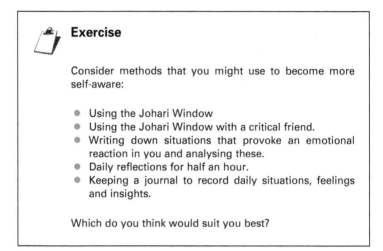

Exercise

Consider methods that you might use to become more self-aware:

- Using the Johari Window
- Using the Johari Window with a critical friend.
- Writing down situations that provoke an emotional reaction in you and analysing these.
- Daily reflections for half an hour.
- Keeping a journal to record daily situations, feelings and insights.

Which do you think would suit you best?

Benefits of self-awareness

In the United Kingdom the NHS (2004) identified self-awareness as one of 15 key components to effective leadership. A high level of self-awareness is believed to sustain the leader's energy and resilience, enabling them to deal with difficult situations. They also suggested that by recognizing their own strengths and limitations mangers are more likely to empower others. They believe that successful leadership and collaborative working requires leaders who are well aware of, and sensitive to, the impact they have on others in a range of work situations (NHS Leadership Centre 2004). While at this point in your career you may not consider yourself a leader, it is important to remember that in many ways everyone has leadership roles. Whether this is role modelling for junior staff or patients or managing a group presentation or assignment, at some point we are called upon to lead. What is also important about this is the importance placed on self-awareness as an aspect of self-development at the highest national level. Similarly public views of a recent review of nurse education provision in the Republic of Ireland were that nurses should be self-aware (Department of Health 2012). Thus, while this may seem an ethereal skill for

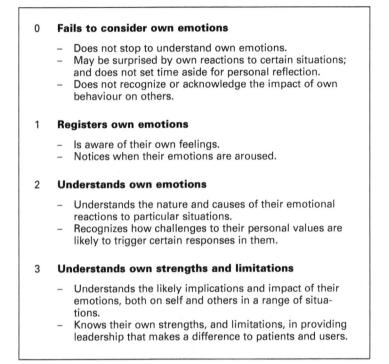

0 **Fails to consider own emotions**

  - Does not stop to understand own emotions.
  - May be surprised by own reactions to certain situations; and does not set time aside for personal reflection.
  - Does not recognize or acknowledge the impact of own behaviour on others.

1 **Registers own emotions**

  - Is aware of their own feelings.
  - Notices when their emotions are aroused.

2 **Understands own emotions**

  - Understands the nature and causes of their emotional reactions to particular situations.
  - Recognizes how challenges to their personal values are likely to trigger certain responses in them.

3 **Understands own strengths and limitations**

  - Understands the likely implications and impact of their emotions, both on self and others in a range of situations.
  - Knows their own strengths, and limitations, in providing leadership that makes a difference to patients and users.

Figure 10.3 NHS Modernisation Agency Leadership Centre Leadership Qualities Framework (LQFR)

Source: NHS Modernization Agency Leadership Centre Leadership Qualities Framework (LQFR); online at www.executive.modern.nhs.uk/framework/personalqualities/selfawareness.aspx Crown Copyright. Reproduced under the Open Government Licence v1.0.

personal use it is one that is crucial to professional development, and viewed as high importance by key stakeholders. An example of this is the National Health Service's NHS development of a tool to use as a measurement scale for assessing personal levels of self-awareness as a component of the leadership qualities framework (LQFR) (NHS Leadership Centre 2004) (Figure 10.3). This is no longer available on this website and is not included in the final report (NHS Leadership Centre 2004).

> **Exercise**
>
> Use Figure 10.3 as a tool to assess your own level of self-awareness.
>   Later ask your critical friend to assess you using the same tool. Compare the results.
>   What have you learned from this experience?

Burnard (1997) also suggests ways in which self-awareness may be important in nursing (Figure 10.4). It must be noted however that these benefits are merely proposed and little empirical research has been carried out in this area. What is of interest in Figure 10.4 is that while self-awareness is a personal journey the professed benefits are primarily to others. There are issues with this. First, there is little evidence confirming that the development of self-awareness can improve performance as little or no experimental work has been carried out on the topic. Second, with an emphasis on highlighting both strengths and weaknesses, there may be a tendency for some to focus upon weaknesses rather than strengths. For example, when nursing students write journals, diaries or reflective pieces of writing there is a tendency to reflect upon negative experiences, as these tend to stand out more, and perhaps the benefit of reflecting upon good experiences is not clear. However, overall, DeVito (2011) suggests that there are several rewards to developing self-awareness including:

- developing self-knowledge,
- improved coping abilities,
- enhanced communication skills, and
- more meaningful relationships.

However DeVito (2011) also reminds us of the risks that come with self-disclosure. You may suffer personal risks by exposing yourself to others, for example in a competitive environment other people having knowledge about you may cause difficulty. You may also risk compromising or losing the relationship (with the critical friend) or run professional risks (for example, disclosing your illegal activity would contravene

Proposed benefits from self-awareness

- Ensuring that people feel cared for
- Understanding other people's needs and wants
- Helping people express their feelings
- Coping with other people's pain
- Helping with people who are dying
- Helping the bereaved
- Working with children
- Learning nursing
- Doing research
- Understanding your colleagues
- Learning to relax
- Getting on better with your friends and family
- Planning your work
- Identifying your strengths and deficits
- Planning your future
- Identifying your learning needs
- Organizing the work of others

Figure 10.4   Proposed benefits from self-awareness

Source: adapted from Burnard, P. (1997) *Know Yourself! Self-Awareness Activities for Nurses and Other Health Professionals*, London: Whurr Publishers Limited.

professional requirements may require your mentor to take relevant action) (DeVito 2011). Ways to avoid these risks is through the careful and appropriate choice of critical friend, careful selective disclosure (which in the case of your nursing programme would be carefully linked to your learning outcomes, rather than anything that randomly comes into your head) and choosing specific situations to discuss that are not overly emotive or personal for you.

Developing self-awareness has become synonymous with reflection, which has gained increasing popularity in nursing over the past 20 years.

Reflection

Reflection is a recurring theme in nursing literature (Hannigan 2001). Based on the work of Dewey (1933), Schön (1983) and others reflection has been an espoused activity in nursing and nurse education in throughout Europe and the United Kingdom (Bulman and Schutz 2008). It is accepted nowadays that nurses should demonstrate critical awareness and reflective practice, thus, learning outcomes related to reflection have become a component part of many undergraduate nurse education programmes and reflection forms the basis for many formative assessments (Hannigan 2001).

Exercise

Why do you think nurses need to be reflective?

Carroll et al. (2002) were critical of both the teaching and assessment of reflection and reflective practice in nursing suggesting that 'the literature on reflection and reflective practice is sparse in terms of research evidence. Large amounts of descriptive anecdotal literature exist, but conclusive answers to the question of what is reflection and how it is to be taught/learned are not apparent'. One concern expressed by these authors was the lack of empirical evidence with regard to improvement in patient outcome through the use of reflection. This argument was supported in a commentary on the paper written by Newell (2002), a seminal author on the topic. Newell supported the argument that reflection may be a topic that is nebulous and not fully articulated or examined, with little purported benefits to patients ultimately emerging. These criticisms need to be borne in mind when considering reflection in the context of practice and the development of reflective practice, which is another concept entirely again not fully elucidated. That said however, there is potential self-development from using the processes of reflection to think back over your actions and to commit to those memories to paper rendering them easier to analyze and thus learn from.

Exercise

How do you think nurses using reflection to develop self-awareness can help patients in their care?

Traditionally, within nursing, reflection has been an individual insular task. However, this may be dependent on purpose. For the purpose of self-development having another person support you in reflection activities is crucial in developing awareness, as you will probably have noticed from the exercises in this chapter. Indeed the notion of reflection has been criticized for being too introspective, and failing to take into account the wider healthcare perspective (Brechin et al. 2000). By focusing solely on what the individual thinks and feels in a given situation there is a tendency towards personal bias and missing out on vital information.

There are several models of reflection on action cited in the literature such as Johns (2009) and Gibbs (1988). These models stimulate reflection after an event has taken place. The focus is on analyzing the situation, exploring feelings, behaviours and reactions and learning from that experience. Strategies used to promote reflection among nursing students include: analysis of critical incidents, diaries and journals (Hannigan 2001). However Jensen and Joy (2005) in their analysis of junior nursing students' journals found very little evidence of reflection taking place, and where it did take place it was mostly at a superficial level. Similarly Timmins and Dunne (2009) found a mostly superficial level of reflection with portfolio use. It is important therefore that you as a student begin to develop skills of deep, honest reflection focusing on yourself [and not others].

While there are professed benefits to using models of reflection, there is little empirical evidence that indicates personal or professional benefits (Carroll et al. 2002). Reflection may be overly introspective (Brechin et al. 2000) and not contain the essential element of feedback from others that is required to develop self-awareness. While personal reflection remains internalized there is always the risk of the use of defence mechanisms and as Burnard (1997) describes these can be used to 'fool' ourselves.

For example, a nursing student may realize through reflection that more communication and explanation could have been afforded to the client during a procedure (intramuscular injection). Although the student admits this, through the course of reflection, the student may use rationalization and intellectualization to provide excuses for the behaviour and thus justify it. The student may decide that little change in the said behaviour is required. As long as reflection remains personal this risk will be there. Alternative solutions are guided reflection as suggested by Johns (1996, 2002) or expanding reflection techniques to encompass critical practice.

Barnett (1997) suggested that inherent domains of critical practice are critical analysis, critical action and critical reflexivity. It is argued that health professionals require all three skills to meet the challenges of a practice that is filled with uncertainty (Brechin et al. 2000). *Critical analysis* requires ongoing enquiry and analysis. Rather than simply relying on prior knowledge and policies, the practitioner *evaluates* their relevance. As opposed to an individualistic perspective, critical analysis recognizes multiple perspectives. *Critical action* requires a sound knowledge base, but seeks to address power differences. *Critical reflexivity* requires a practitioner who is self-aware in his/her practice. Critical practice is viewed as a process. Further exploration of these domains process serves to illuminate the potential contribution of these concepts to nursing practice.

Critical analysis

Critical practice is represented by an overlap of critical analysis, critical action and critical reflexivity (Barnett 1997). The specific components of critical analysis are outlined in Figure 10.5.

Using critical analysis can encourage nurses to question their practice. They will begin to examine inherent strengths and weaknesses of their practice. They will also evaluate their current knowledge and theory. This analysis will be continuous and ongoing and occur at multiple levels including at the personal level. The nurse will continuously question his/her own knowledge and theory base to evaluate the extent to which it informs current practice.

Increasingly the nursing profession is also being called upon to recognize different perspectives. Modern healthcare strategies require a people-centred approach, where the

Evaluation of knowledge, theories, policy, and practice

Recognition of multiple perspectives

Different levels of analysis

Ongoing enquiry

Figure 10.5   Critical analysis

Source: adapted from Brechin, A. (2000) Introducing critical practice. In A. Brechin, H. Brown and M. Eby (eds), *Critical Practice in Health and Social Care*, London: Sage Publications, 25–47.

consumer (i.e., the patient) is placed at the centre of health-care rather than nursing priorities as the centre of care. Critical analysis encourages nurses to see the patient's perspective.

Critical action

The key features of critical action are outlined in Figure 10.6. Critical practice also requires a solid skill base. Critical action requires empowering the nursing profession from within. Improving knowledge and skills through continuous education and development is one element. Empowerment of patients also involves tackling some of the oppression that exists within society towards marginalized groups (Pinkery 2000).

Sound skill base used with awareness of context

Operating to challenge structural disadvantage

Working with difference towards empowerment

Figure 10.6   Critical action

Source: adapted from Brechin, A. (2000) Introducing critical practice. In A. Brechin, H. Brown and M. Eby (eds), *Critical Practice in Health and Social Care*, London: Sage Publications, 25–47.

Critical reflexivity

The impetus for, and the origin of, both critical analysis and critical action are largely outside the individual (Brechin et al. 2000). The professional role and the organization provide an incentive and a platform for these activities, and indeed a certain responsibility exists therein. However, the third aspect of critical practice, critical reflexivity, is inherently personal. The key features of critical reflexivity are described briefly in Figure 10.7. Reflexivity is a particularly useful strategy for developing self-awareness. Critical reflexivity provides direction for nurses to think about practice. While reflection in isolation has been criticized for being too individualistic within healthcare delivery, critical reflexivity within the context of critical practice is not. Nash's (2000) reflection on practice provides an example of the limitations. While this was useful to her personally, there was little evidence that it would inform policy on a wider level or that it considered wider contributions. With critical practice, however, the findings induced through critical reflexivity inform critical action and analysis and contribute to the overall understanding of a situation. The guiding principles of critical practice are: 'respecting others as equals' and 'adopting a not all-knowing approach' (Brechin et al. 2000: 31). Analyzing policy, challenging oppression and introspection must be done with respect. The approach should be objective. Adopting a 'not all-knowing' approach is the only feasible option open to today's nurses and practitioners. An example of how this critical reflexivity may be used to develop self-awareness follows.

Engaged self
Negotiated understanding and interventions
Questioning personal values and assumptions

Figure 10.7 Critical reflexivity

Source: adapted from Brechin, A. (2000) Introducing critical practice. In A. Brechin, H. Brown and M. Eby (eds), *Critical Practice in Health and Social Care*, London: Sage Publications, 25–47.

Example: a case study

During your recent placement in a large nursing home you look after an 86 year old widow named Marjorie Peabody, a retired school teacher who had recently sold her home and come to live full-time in the nursing home. She was quite independent with her daily activities up until her admission, although her mobility was somewhat limited somewhat due to a previous history of a hip replacement and angina.

During your first day or two in the home you notice how nice and homely Marjorie's room looks as she has brought with her a lot of her own furniture. There are lots of photographs of her when she was younger with her husband who was a pilot. She had travelled with him extensively and from all the books in her room you could see that she was an avid reader.

In your journal one evening you are writing down your daily events and speak about assisting her one day with her hygiene. You had felt under pressure and rushed to complete this task, and had overheard some of the staff talking about how 'slow' it was to get her ready in the morning and how 'fussy' she was about doing her hair and make-up. You are keen to do well on this placement and were thinking out ways of speeding things up the next day, while at the same time maintaining good communication when it struck you that this really was not the best approach. Using the critical practice framework, you analyzed the case in your journal over the coming week (anonymously).

Step 1 Critical analysis (see Figure 10.5)

- You researched about hygiene policies and person-centred care approaches.
- You observed the practice of various nurses with patients.
- You talked to nurses and your tutors about providing hygiene care for this patient group.

- You revisited your classroom notes, textbooks and found published research papers on the topic.

Step 2 Critical action (see Figure 10.6)

- Following on from step 1 you become determined to provide holistic patient-centred care that encourages Marjorie's independence and reduces her vulnerability.
- You avoid *doing for* Marjorie things that she could easily, and certainly liked to, do herself.
- You focus on getting to know Marjorie more and referring to her photos when you are with her in order to maintain her dignity, personhood and individuality.
- You work closely with and seek advice from qualified staff on the matter.
- You try to remain aware of the particular context (the busy nursing home) and your own role and requirements within.

Step 3 Critical reflexivity (see Figure 10.7)

- You engage yourself wholeheartedly in your actions in a humanistic honest way.
- When considering the context you ascertain whether or not your 'actions' are suitable to the environment. Is there a better way of doing things? For example, your actions may considerably slow down the work of the organization, is this something (on negotiation) that could be done at a different time or alternative days?
- You adopt an open, not all-knowing approach. Don't think that you are necessarily right, keep an open mind, talk to others [including the client] and remember that you have personal values and assumptions that effect your actions. Question whether any of your assumptions come into play here. Did you assume that Marjorie wished to have long chats about her travels/husband simply because this is your experience of older people? Did you ask her?

You will see from this case study that developing self-awareness is not only something that can be done by personal introspection but something that you can link to your practice to develop yourself as an emerging practitioner. When considering situations to examine or write about in your diary remember never to mention patient names or revealing patient details. Try to avoid, especially in the beginning, seeking out crisis situations [where you or other staff were very emotional for example] as it is unlikely that you have the skills to deal with these complex situations. Keep it simple and try to examine and reflect upon the ordinary aspects of your own personal nursing practice. You will also see from this study that it is almost impossible to analyze your communication skills without examining your skills as a nurse in the delivery of patient care. This is an important finding, as communication in the healthcare setting does not occur in a vacuum and is often part and parcel of our actions on a daily basis (McCabe 2004), thus reflections on communications should be done with this in mind. Furthermore while some communications take place on a one-to-one basis, many occur in the presence of other members of the multidisciplinary team, family or other patients. Thus, detailed critical reflection on your actions and communications is required on an ongoing basis to clearly examine your role and effect in this complex system.

Developing professional confidence

Bandura (1986) wrote that, through the process of self-reflection, individuals are able to evaluate their experiences and thought processes. According to this view, what people know, the skills they possess, or what they have previously accomplished are not always good predictors of subsequent attainments because the beliefs they hold about their capabilities powerfully influence the ways in which they will behave. Consequently, how people behave is both mediated by their beliefs about their capabilities and can often be predicted better by these beliefs than by the results of their previous performances. Thus, reflection alone is not sufficient to improve performance. It could indeed have a negative effect. A supportive environment with the use of a facilitator is therefore very helpful, and indeed recommended (Johns 1996) in the development of future confidence with nursing skills when using self-awareness/reflective techniques. Nursing students therefore should, where possible, aim to develop self-awareness skills under the guidance of a critical friend and nursing facilitator, preceptor, mentor, teacher or guide as appropriate.

This is especially important as the discussion of self-awareness within the nursing context focuses upon the recognition of personal strengths and weakness. To a certain extent the personal weaknesses are the focus of scrutiny as you seek to improve behaviour that will ultimately improve the therapeutic relationship. The impact of you uncovering these negative aspects can affect your confidence, and therefore it is useful to talk through these things with a nurse whom you can trust. Sometimes nursing students are a little fearful of this, but it is important to remember your responsibility to the organization/university/profession. As a growing professional it is incumbent upon you to develop your communication skills in this way. You are developing your skills for the public in a very public way, supported by public organizations. While this does not mean you need to divulge your hidden self to all and sundry it does mean that you ought not to be afraid of selective reflection/developing self-awareness with the aid of a mentor that you can trust.

In the absence of reflection that is guided or supervised by a critical friend or mentor, you run the risk applying your own defence mechanisms during reflection (rationalization, intellectualization, projection, reaction formation, suppression, repression, regression) or conversely actually internalizing negative findings that could possibly reduce confidence. The use of a professional guide, such as a counsellor or mentor would reduce this risk as the person could be coached away from this line of thinking. Your guide might also advise you on situations that they might consider more suitable for your self-development.

Exercise

Imagine you underwent several bladder operations as a child and were hospitalized for several months. You still have some ongoing minor problems and occasional infections.

Your next placement is on a children's ward, so as part of your reflections you decide to examine your communications with the family of one child who is admitted for bladder surgery.

There have been major developments in the surgery since your own hospital experience and the child is to be discharged within 24 hours of admission.

You notice from your diary that you have written six pages about the case, and you are extremely sympathetic towards the family. You are determined to act on this sympathy the following shift.

Consider:

Is this the most apt case to build your self-awareness with?
What reasons would you consider it not to be a suitable case?
What reasons would you give to suggest that it is a suitable case?
You will see that this is a most superficial reflection. It pertains to what you saw on the ward and your experiences/feelings. Do you think that it is appropriate to plan actions based on this?
Do you think a more critical analysis is needed (looking at knowledge/policy in the area)?
Do you think a more critical reflexivity is needed (considering your own assumptions)?
Do you believe that having a mentor or critical friend to guide you in this reflection or towards another reflection would be useful?

Hopefully from this exercise you will have learnt the potential benefit of working with another person in the development of your self-awareness. In this situation, for example, if you became upset it might be helpful to have someone with you, as you are delving in to a very personal area of your life. You will also see the limitations of superficial reflection. In this case you only had your daily experience and your past experience to guide your actions, and this is not the best method (although it occurs commonly) of reflection. You may have pointed out that examining your textbooks, articles and ward materials would give you a good understanding of the child's operation (not your own view of it from experience). Similarly seeking out the child/families' views (rather than basing it on your own assumptions) would be best. Finally beginning by seeking the advice of a mentor may have resulted in you picking a rather more ordinary topic that would be of equal benefit to your development [and less emotive, time-consuming and misleading] such as family-centred care in relation to preoperative preparation of children.

Here we are using self-awareness to build and develop professional confidence rather than using it to gather information about possible misguided actions, which appears to be the default option. Unlike self-awareness and reflection, the concept of confidence is something that has undergone significant theoretical and empirical development under the guidance of Bandura (1977).

Bandura (1977) introduced the term self-efficacy as the belief that one can execute a specific activity successfully. Expectations of personal efficacy are based on four major sources of information: performance accomplishments, vicarious experience, verbal persuasion, and physiological state. 'Self-confidence is the feeling that someone knows how to do something, has the power to make things happen, and knows that one's efforts will be successful; it is the belief that knowledge, skill, experience, and potential will result in success' (Davidhizar 1993: 218).

According to Bandura (1997) self-efficacy makes a difference to how people feel, think and act. For example, a low sense of self-efficacy is associated with depression, anxiety and helplessness (Scholz et al. 2002). This may result in low self-esteem and negative views of one's personal accomplishments and personal development. Conversely, a high self-efficacy improves performance including that of decision-making and academic achievement (Scholz et al. 2002). Therefore self-efficacy levels can increase or reduce motivation. People with high self-efficacy choose to perform more challenging tasks (Bandura 1997). They often set high goals that they are determined to achieve (Schwarzer and Schmitz 2004). High self-efficacy also allows people to recover more quickly from setbacks that occur, therefore, maintaining commitment to their original goals. Thus, self-efficacy allows individuals to explore and responds to challenging environments (Scholz et al. 2002).

Scholz et al. (2002) suggested that self-efficacy is 'domain-specific'. This means that firm self-beliefs can be held in particular situations of functioning. But some researchers have also conceptualized a generalized sense of self-efficacy that refers to a global confidence in one's coping ability across a wide range of demanding or novel situations. General self-efficacy aims at a broad and stable sense of personal competence to deal effectively with a variety of stressful situations. According to Bandura's (1986) social cognitive theory, individuals possess a self-system that enables them to exercise a measure of control over their thoughts, feelings, motivation and actions. This self-system provides reference mechanisms and a set of sub functions for perceiving, regulating, and evaluating behaviour, which results from the interplay between the system and environmental sources of influence. As such, it serves a self-regulatory function by providing individuals with the capability to influence their own cognitive processes and actions and thus alter their environments.

How people interpret the results of their own performance attainments informs and alters their environments and their self-beliefs which, in turn, inform and alter subsequent performance. In general, Bandura provided a view of human behaviour in which the beliefs that people have about themselves are key elements in the exercise of control and personal agency and in which individuals are viewed both as products and as producers of their own environments and of their social systems.

Conclusion

This chapter considered the meaning of self-awareness in the context of contemporary healthcare and outlines ways to develop and improve self-awareness. Some time was spent considering the meaning of self-awareness. Freud proposed the notion of the unconscious self. The humanistic model pays greater attention to self-awareness. Humans are motivated towards continual self-improvement. Peplau (1991) described how the self develops from appraisals made by self and significant others as an infant and child. Burnard (1997) provided a simple model of the self. Developing self-awareness has an important role in enhancing self-understanding, self monitoring and can be useful in nursing situations.

Reflection is gaining increasing popularity within the nursing profession. Burnard (1985, 1997), a key author in this area, highlighted the increased development of self-awareness as a positive element in nurses and a requirement of professional nursing practice. Through developing a greater awareness of self, elements of self can be explored and developed in order to improve communication skills (Burnard 1997). Through self-awareness and recognition of emotions valuable information can be learned. Barnett's (1997) domains of critical practice (critical analysis, critical action and critical reflexivity) were explored and applied to the practice of self-awareness. Critical analysis, critical action and critical reflexivity are considered essential factors in developing professional self-awareness. Reflexivity is a particularly useful skill for developing self-awareness in nurses. Critical reflexivity provides direction for nurses to think about practice. Self-awareness is an essential ingredient in the development of effective patient-centred communication.

Key points

- ▶ Self-awareness is an essential ingredient in the development of effective patient-centred communication. It is also essential for the persona, and therefore professional growth and development.
- ▶ Self-awareness is about knowing and understanding ourselves and without it we cannot begin to understand others.
- ▶ Developing self-awareness requires that our feelings, actions, values attitudes and beliefs are brought into our consciousness and we become aware of how we as individuals and nurses influence our relationships and interactions with others.
- ▶ Critical analysis, critical action and critical reflexivity are considered essential factors in developing professional self-awareness and are key components of critical practice.

11 Experiential Learning

Introduction

Securing and practicing from a uniform knowledge base is essential to the development of the discipline of nursing. It is widely recognized and accepted that nursing practice must be based on research. Internationally, the use of research in nursing is regarded as a necessary step in an age of continued rapid technological development and quality care. Increasingly, practitioners are called upon to justify their practice and ensure that it is based on sound evidence. What constitutes evidence attracts debate within the nursing domain and research is an accepted and legitimate source of evidence that is essential for many aspects of nursing care.

However, the research base for nurse–patient communication and the development of the therapeutic relationship with clients is not well established. While textbooks on communication abound, most of the work is prescriptive and descriptive, thus describing models of communication and outlining how nurses in practice may use these. As outlined in Chapter 1, many of these conceptual models fail to fully account for the complexity of the communication process, and although these models may be useful for developing an understanding of aspects of communication they provide little by way of direction for nurse–patient communication in the clinical setting. Although they serve to provide some explanation for communication events they are abstract and removed from the dynamic interaction of communication within the therapeutic relationship. Chapter 1 also highlighted how few of these theories are specific to nursing. Morse et al. (1992), in a widely referred to seminal piece of work, developed a model of communication that focuses on the emotional engagement of the nurse with the patient (Figure 1.2). The model is based on two key characteristics. The first is whether the nurse is patient-focused or nurse-focused and the second is whether the communication is spontaneous (first-level) or learned (second-level). Fosbinder (1994) revealed that important aspects of communication from a patient's perspective were translating, getting to know you, establishing trust and going the extra mile. Morse et al. (1992) also highlighted the importance of the display of sympathy by nurses to patients McCabe's (2004) study supported this.

Morse et al. (1997) developed the Comforting Interaction-Relationship Model and identified three components of communication: nursing actions, patient actions and the evolving relationship. Nursing actions consist of comforting strategies, styles of care and nursing patterns of relating. Patient actions consist of signals of discomfort, indices of distress and patterns of relating to a nurse. The evolving relationship is the third component of this model and it describes nursing and patient actions as the means by which the nurse–patient relationship is negotiated by the nurse and patient and subsequently develops. Nurses respond to patient signals of discomfort and indices of distress using comforting strategies, styles of caring and patterns of relating on an ongoing and changing basis.

Nurses often use a linear model of one-way communication in the practice setting (sender-message-receiver) that limits communication and the development of the nurse–patient relationship (Kruijver et al. 2001). It is suggested that using the *principles* of good communication, such as those suggested by Morse et al. (1997), rather than the static models of communication results in more effective patient–centred communication.

A further notion is the development and exploration of nursing knowledge using interpretive approaches (Benner et al. 1999; Benner 2000). Benner's aforementioned seminal and influential work guided critical care nurses away from using frameworks that involved listing diagnoses and matching interventions, (static models) towards the practice of using clinical judgment. As an alternative, these authors suggest that critical care nurses should focus on six aspects of clinical judgment and skilful behaviour: (1) reasoning-in-transition; (2) skilled knowledge; (3) response-based practice; (4) agency; (5) perceptual ability and the skill of involvement; and (6) the links between clinical and ethical reasoning. These aspects of practice may serve as a guide for use to articulate nursing care for documentation and teaching and improving practice (Benner et al. 1999).

A similar approach could be used with communication. Nursing actions (comforting strategies, styles of care and nursing patterns of relating) described by Morse et al. (1992) could be used as a framework to develop a repertoire of communication skills. Through ongoing reflection on practice, including feedback from both clients and peer's nursing actions, patient actions and the evolving relationship could be articulated. Rather than expecting a communication model or theory to fully inform practice, the nurse may develop a dynamic theory through critical practice. This complies with other influential authors such as Watson (1999, n.d.) who articulated the notion of a Science of Caring that embraces 'inquiries that are reflective, subjective and interpretative as well as objective-empirical' (Watson 2005). Watson (2005) suggested that this caring science served as an 'intellectual blueprint for nursing's evolving disciplinary/professional matrix, rather than a specific theory per sé'. To this end it is useful to incorporate some of her seminal principles here.

Watson (2005) advocates multiple approaches to inquiry and theory building including clinical and empirical, but was also open to moving other areas of inquiry such as the aesthetic, poetic and narratives. Thus, in a postmodern era, there is a place for building on theory using reflection, narratives, personal enquiry and experiential learning.

Methods of experiential learning in communication

Communication with patients and clients takes place in many environments: hospital wards, clinics, nursing homes and clients' own homes. The nursing student, although equipped with the relevant classroom preparation and theory is likely to learn a great deal about communication through a variety of experiences. In order to draw out specific learning from those experiences it may be helpful to begin to write up a daily journal or diary, or simply write about critical incidents, those interactions that may have struck you as important in some way during the day. Diaries are often used in nursing and are mostly for the personal use of the student. Writing is free from restrictions and is a personal narrative however, to preserve confidentiality of patients and clients, names and other identifiable characteristics should be avoided when making references to practice. Security of the diary/journal is also important, and it should be kept in a safe and private place at all times. This journal or diary is a narrative giving a descriptive account of experiences of the practice of nursing. It may be useful for articulating and clarifying thoughts and facilitate the development of questions about practice that may be investigated through the course of study or by subsequently asking questions of a mentor/preceptor or staff nurse.

Example

Julie is a first year student nurse working on a cardiac ward. She begins writing her diary on her first day of the placement on the ward and writes it up each evening. She has been on the ward for four weeks and is getting used to performing in this environment. However, she realized from writing her diary that there are still several items in the morning report/ handover that she does not understand. This relates particularly to abbreviations used by staff. She decides to ask a member of staff to talk through the report with her during a quiet period the following day.

This example demonstrates how simple description of the day's activities revealed an item that Julie needed to address. This type of work is personal and superficial. In order to deepen the level of analysis the use of a model of reflection such as Gibbs (1988) may be used.

Using a model of reflection

Using a model of reflection such as Gibbs (1988) provides a little more structure than a diary or journal. Although now dated, this model is commonly used by undergraduate nursing students (Rolfe et al. 2011; O'Donovan 2006). It provides specific guidelines for the thought processes. This can be used on a specific topic or incident being discussed within a diary or journal or it can be performed as an isolated reflection exercise. It is important to remember too that reflecting on ordinary everyday nursing situations also yields very powerful and important learning (Benner 2000). Benner's (2000) categories for critical incidents in nursing are:

- Those in which your interventions really made a difference.
- Those that went unusually well.
- Those in which there was a breakdown.
- Those that were ordinary and typical.
- Those that captured the essence of nursing.
- Those that were particularly demanding.

It is useful to use the steps of the cycle of reflection as subheadings to describe and analyze the situation. The subheadings are outlined in Figure 11.1.

Steps in Reflection

- Description: what happened?
- Feelings: what were you thinking/feeling?
- Evaluation: what was good and bad about the experience?
- Conclusion: what else would you have done?
- Analysis: what sense can you make of the situation?
- Action Plan: if it arose again what would you do?

Figure 11.1   Steps in the reflection process

Source: adapted from Gibbs, G., Palmer, A., Burns, S. and Bulman, C. (1994) *Reflective Practice in Nursing*, Oxford: Blackwell Scientific Publications.

An example of a reflection is outlined below.

Description: what happened?
On the ward today I was asked whether I would like to give an injection to a patient. I had seen it being given before but had not done one yet.

Feelings: what were you thinking/feeling?
I was delighted that I was getting a chance to do it. They do not come up that often on this ward

Evaluation: what was good and bad about the experience?
The staff nurse who supervised me explained everything in advance and that was great. I really felt confident when I began. I gave the injection pretty well I think, the nurse said that I had done well.

Conclusion: what else would you have done?
Although actually giving the injection went well, I do not think that I focused enough on the patient. The nurse did all the talking and explaining as I was so focused on what I was doing. Looking back on it, I could have explained things more to the patient and involved her a little more.

Analysis: what sense can you make of the situation?
I mentioned these thoughts to the nurse afterwards, and she explained that as I was a junior student, and it was my first time, this was not unusual. I agree with this, it was very difficult to come to grips with holding all the equipment, positioning myself and trying to explain things to the patient at the same time. I suppose this will improve with time.

Action plan: if it arose again what would you do?
Definitely, even as a junior student I would make a bigger effort to provide explanations to the patient.

Using a model such as Gibbs (1988) provides structure and guidelines for reflection and can guide the student towards future action in the area. Criticisms of model use include the tendency for students to focus on negative aspects of their practice, or to search for negative aspects. This may be as a result of the subheadings that while useful, are also leading. The last section for example 'what would do if it arose again?', and 'what else could you have done?' may lead the student to look for situations where action is needed (as opposed to no action being required). There is also a tendency for this type of reflection to be self-limiting. It is a superficial analysis of subjective feelings and it is unclear whether this is useful or meaningful to students or whether (as described in Chapter 10) it has any overall impact upon nursing practice.

One method of advancing reflection and experiential learning is critical practice (Chapter 10). Critical practice, while alluded to many texts, is not always sufficiently unpacked to allow the reader a full understanding of how to take it forward into practice. Barnett's (1997) unique approach provides an excellent explanation of how critical practice works. Rather than providing an introspective analysis, critical practice encourages feedback from others and consideration of the context in which the practice of nursing takes place. Key components of critical practice are critical analysis critical, action and critical reflexivity (Barnett 1997).

Critical analysis requires ongoing enquiry and analysis. Rather than simply relying on prior knowledge and policies, the practitioner *evaluates* their relevance. Using the example of the administration of an intramuscular injection above, the student when engaging in critical analysis would not only explore personal feelings and behaviours but move outside of this personal realm to examine carefully personal knowledge related to the procedure. Rather than reflection on action or in action this analysis may be done prior to the procedure to inform subsequent practice. This may involve examining notes from the classroom, textbooks, ward policies and observation of practice and recording these in the journal.

Critical analysis also encourages the recognition of multiple perspectives. Very often students focus on discrepancies between their received teaching and the practice observed on the wards. In their reflection these observations can thwart their perception of their learning experience guided perhaps by a belief in 'perfectionism' as articulated by Watson (1999: 37) who suggested that nursing students are 'led to believe that only perfect practice is permissible in clinical areas'. This is not to suggest that best practice or evidence-based practice is not adhered to, but rather refers to the observation by students of expert practice as described by Benner et al. (1999) that deviates slightly from the mechanized procedure that a student has been taught.

One such procedure may be patient hygiene. The nurse may not have attended to hygiene needs in the particular order and sequence taught to the student in the classroom and this may be a cause for concern to the student. Critical analysis of situations encourages the student to explore multiple perspectives. A non-judgemental student-led discussion after observing the procedure is required so that the student may understand the perspective of the nurse and this would be a good learning experience. There may be a very clear rationale for this deviation in procedure. It could be that the ward policy is different to that taught in the classroom. Or there may be other reasons. Whatever the justification, the idea is that the students explore the multiple facets of the situation rather than relying solely on personal reflection and introspection that may be of limited value particularly for junior students who often report that they do not really know what they are reflecting upon.

Using the example of intramuscular injection, the student may have observed the procedure and rather than moving straight to performance under supervision it may have been useful to have a discussion with the teacher or mentor to gain more insight into their perspective. In addition to elucidating any perceived discrepancies the student may learn the subtleties of expert practice as the nurse begins to articulate those aspects of practice not necessarily accounted for in the procedure, such as a gentle touch of the hand during explanation.

Critical analysis also involves different levels of analysis. This implies not only personal analysis and consideration of personal actions required in a situation, but an analysis of the context (the ward, the patient, the atmosphere, the relationships), ward policy and procedures, other people's views of the situation and the client's view. This type of analysis discourages the introspection of reflection that solely encourages the analysis of personal feelings in situations. The context in which interactions take place is crucial to our understanding of events. Brechin et al. (2000), who applied many of Barnett's (1997) guiding principles to health and social care, suggested that this analysis should be ongoing, so rather than leaving analysis as single entries in a journal they would feed into others and develop as a theme throughout the journal.

Another vehicle for the collection of such information that is gaining increasing popularity in nursing is a portfolio (Scholes et al. 2004). These authors describe a portfolio as a 'purposeful collection of traditional and non-traditional work that represents a student's learning, progress and achievement over time'. Reflection commonly forms part of a portfolio, and the portfolio may be used as part components of course work assessment. The portfolio is particularly useful for outlining particular themes that can be developed. When applying a critical analysis framework the portfolio can be useful for storing the relevant information.

The next component of critical practice is critical action. Brechin et al. (2000) suggested that one should operate with a sound skill base used with an awareness of context. Having performed the necessary analysis in the first part of this cycle the student will have gained increased knowledge about the skill from analyzing prior learning, ward procedures and through discussions with others. It is also suggested that the student operates to challenge structural disadvantage and works with difference towards empowerment that present a challenge for students at a junior level. However, it is worth reading, reflecting and observing these skills, and writing about them within the portfolio, as these skills are crucial to modern nursing. Contemporary notions of health and healthcare are based on patient empowerment and reduction of disadvantage, so the student must begin to consider these in their practice. Using the example of the intramuscular injection, patient empowerment may simply involve providing choice as to whether a student may perform the procedure. Although it may seem pedantic, it is the beginnings of recognizing patients as equal partners in care and not passive recipients of care.

After the procedure the patient's views may be elicited and this too would provide a level of patient involvement and empowerment.

The final section in the critical practice cycle is critical reflexivity. While this is the inherently personal aspect of critical practice, it involves less introspection. The student is encouraged to become engaged with practice, consider practice issues and also to negotiate understandings. Rather than the student operating from a one-sided perspective they are encouraged to share their understanding of situations and listen to other's views to inform their view. It is also suggested that one questions personal values and assumptions. So that rather than operating from the 'perfectionist' stance, as articulated by Watson (1999), values and beliefs are continually being questioned. Figures 11.2 and 11.3 are two examples of portfolio entries. Note elements of critical practice as you read.

You may have noticed that that policies and current practice were taken into consideration in both entries. The use of a textbook indicated the development of a sound knowledge base. At times the writer was attempting to work towards reducing disadvantage by considering gaps in current practice. There was also an attempt towards greater patient empowerment. Ultimately critical reflexivity was present as the writer challenged their own assumptions and came to new understandings about communication practice.

Aspects of communication such as patient action, nursing action and the evolving relationship can be framed within the critical practice framework (Figure 11.4). Fundamental communication skills can be explored, developed and utilized in practice by nursing students and nurses through skills of self-awareness and reflection. This may involve experiential learning documented in diaries, journals or portfolio. Critical analysis can reveal the patient actions and perspective and reveal the specific context for nursing action. Critical action involves empowerment patients through comforting strategies styles of care and relating to patients. Critical reflexivity examines the effectiveness and development of communication through self-engagement, challenging personal assumptions and establishing the extent to which a therapeutic

Portfolio entry 1   Communication skills

During portfolio activity 1, I reflected upon different types of personal communication. The exploration of the communication theories and methods provided valuable additional insight into my own behaviour in this area. I was aware that I was talkative in social situations, and I considered my communication to be of satisfactory standard. The activities and reflection that I undertook during this clinical placement challenged this assumption.

This involved a critical analysis of my listening skills. It became apparent that my listening skills were poor. Whilst I often feigned this skill, in reality I let my mind wander. Such lack of engagements now strikes me as an obvious flaw. It is an essential prerequisite to attending. Clearly, its absence was a barrier to my development as a communicator.

My approach to communication in general deviated towards a person-centred approach (Sidell, 2000). However, empathy, unconditional positive regard and genuineness are crucial to this humanistic style, which in effect were absent on many occasions during that week, when I failed to listen or talked too much. I realised that in order to develop an atmosphere of trust and respect with clients or students, I needed to be a good listener. I also understood that listening is crucial to success in health education situations (see article). I became aware that reasons existed for my failure to listen (Sidell, 2000), which was mainly self-consciousness, although sometimes I just wanted to be the one doing all the talking.

During the week, I was acutely aware of daydreaming when people spoke. This new awareness, prompted by this activity, meant that I began to make a conscious effort to actually listen and attend. I found that while this took effort for the first few minutes, once I made a real effort to listen and move beyond the level basic levels of listening (Sidell, 2000), it became really easy and enjoyable.

Effective communication is a crucial component of effective nursing practice that I now aspire to. I am embarrassed to think that I have been such a poor listener and I hope that the insight that I gained from this portfolio exercise will continue to improve my listening skills and that they will become imbedded in my practice over time. This activity focused and developed personal skills that are useful to practice.

Figure 11.2   Example of a portfolio entry (1)

relationship development and whether the communication was patient centred.

Although theory and models serve to inform communication in the healthcare context, in a post-modern era technical rationality is replaced with a more dynamic model for practice that evolves through experiential learning, critical practice and patient involvement. If the ultimate aim of nurse–patient

---

Portfolio entry 2   Communication in Health Promotion

Learning about myself as a health promoter really took me by surprise. Rather than being merely a learning exercise, the portfolio and other activities encouraged me to review and critically assess my practice. My self-awareness grew through the exploration and justification of my own definition of health and health promotion in the portfolio. I was quite surprised that my notion of health and health promotion was firmly enshrined in the medical model of health. I considered myself already knowledgeable in this area, and I was shocked at how short sighted I had been. My practice was similar to health education (one to one and information giving) as opposed to health promotion (the total needs).

In this activity I critically reviewed and developed my ideas about my approach to health promotion. I was quite amazed to see it described as 'authoritative'. I began to understand the influences on my thinking. Local policy guided my practice. In addition the lifestyle approach, had both national and international approval (Jones, 2000a) and reflected a local response to national targets. My fellow students had a similar approach.

I thought that I had a holistic approach to nursing care as a third year student but I had not translated this holism into my personal thinking and practice in relation to health promotion. On one level, I was obviously aware of the existence of social issues, but had never considered their impact on health. I came to realise during this ward placement that health promotion should be holistic, addressing social and economic inequalities. Reflecting collective, rather than individual intervention. This learning was endorsed through discussion with my mentor.

I developed an increased understanding of the social and economic determinants of health and explored different models of health promotion (Jones 2000a). The consideration of my own beliefs about health was new to me and very enlightening. I realised that people's attitudes and actions towards health are value bound. The limits of a medical approach became apparent to me and I developed a new way of thinking about health, I became willing to move away from a lifestyle (persuasive/individualistic) approach, realizing that it was 'victim blaming'.

I began to align my thinking with changing priorities in health promotion (Jones 2000a), where health is conceptualized as a state of not just freedom from illness, but of psychological and social well-being. This latter aspect of health was illuminated in Cox et al's work (1997, cited in Jones, 2006b). This latter information astounded me. For the future, I decided that my practice would be guided by the values of the Ottawa charter social justice, participation, equity, and empowerment and reflect a less conservative and more collective approach. I was at odds with contemporary health promotion theory and practice. I realized that my approach to health promotion needed to be multi-strategy. Thus I began fundamental changes in my definitions of health and health promotion, and, the next activity, challenged the practice.

Figure 11.3   Example of a portfolio entry (2)

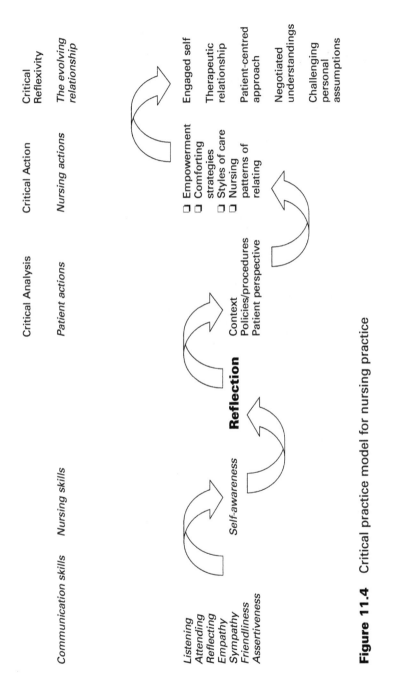

Figure 11.4 Critical practice model for nursing practice

communication is patient centredness then the conceptual models guiding care must also reflect this approach. It is no longer acceptable to continue with a narcissist approach such as reflection. Experiential learning in the healthcare context requires the development of a sound knowledge base, awareness of context, inclusion of patient views, feedback from mentors and the challenging of personal assumptions. All these are features of a critical practice that is suggested as a way forward for the development of the science of communication.

Key points

▶ An eclectic use of models is regarded as effective and useful for explaining and developing nursing practice.

▶ Methods of learning how to communicate positively and effectively with patients include the use of diaries, journals, reflection and the Critical Practice Model. This model consists of three key components, critical analysis, critical action and critical reflexivity and is regarded as a way forward for the development of the science of communication.

▶ Unlike some models of learning, experiential learning reflects the ultimate aim of nurse–patient communication, which is patient centredness

References

Chapter 1

Attree, M. (2001) Patients' and relatives' experiences and perspectives of 'good' and 'not so good' quality care. *Journal of Advanced Nursing*, 33: 456–66.

Balzer-Riley, J. (2011) *Communication in Nursing*, 7th edn (St. Louis, MO: Mosby).

Bateson, G. (1979) *Mind and Nature* (New York: Dutton).

Berlo, D. (1960) *The Process of Communication: An Introduction to the Theory and Practice* (New York: Holt, Rinehart & Winston).

Berry, J.A. (2009) Nurse practitioner/patient communication styles in clinical practice. *The Journal for Nurse Practitioners*, 5(7): 508–15.

Chan, E.A., Jones, A., Fung, S. and Wu Chou, S. (2012) Nurses' perceptions of time availability in patient communication in Hong Kong. *Journal of Clinical Nursing*, 21(7–8): 1168–77.

Craig, R.T. (2001) Communication. In Sloane, T. (ed.) *Encyclopedia of Rhetoric* (New York: Oxford University Press).

DeVito, J.A. (2000) *Human Communication: The Basic Course* (New York: Longman).

DeVito, J.A. (2011) *Essentials of Human Communication*, 7th edn (London: Pearson).

Fosbinder, D. (1994) Patient perceptions of nursing care: An emerging theory of interpersonal competence. *Journal of Advanced Nursing*, 20: 1085–93.

Hargie, O. (2006) Skill in practice: An operational model of communicative skilled performance. In Hargie, O. (ed.) *The Handbook of Communication Skills*, 3rd edn (London: Routledge).

Hargie, O. (2011) *Skilled Interpersonal Communication* (Routledge, London).

Harms, L. (2007) *Working with People: Communication Skills for Reflective Practice* (South Melbourne: Oxford University Press).

Hayes, J. (1991) *Interpersonal Skills: Goal-Directed Behaviour at Work* (London: Harper Collins).

Jakobsson, L. and Holmberg, L. (2012) Quality from the patient's perspective: A one-year trial. *International Journal of Health Care Quality Assurance*, 25(3): 177–88.

Kruijver, J.P.M., Kerkstra, A., Bensing, J.M. and Van de Wiel, H.B.M. (2001) Communication skills of nurses during interactions with simulated cancer patients. *Journal of Advanced Nursing*, 34, 6: 772–9.

McCabe, C. (2004) Nurse-patient communication: An exploration of patients' experiences. *Journal of Clinical Nursing*, 13: 41–9.

McQueen, A. (2000) Nurse-patient relationships and partnership in hospital care. *Journal of Clinical Nursing*, 9: 723–31.

Miller, G.R. and Nicholson, H.E. (1976) *Communication Inquiry: A Perspective on Process*. (Reading: Addison-Wesley).

Morse, J., Bottorff, J., Anderson, G., O'Brien, B. and Solberg, S. (1992) Beyond empathy: expanding expressions of caring. *Journal of Advanced Nursing*, 17: 809–21.

Morse, J.M., De Luca Havens, G.A. and Wilson, S. (1997) The comforting interaction: Developing a model of nurse-patient relationship. *Scholarly Inquiry for Nursing Practice*, 11(4): 321–43.

Peplau, H.E. (1952) *Interpersonal Relations in Nursing: A Conceptual Frame of Reference for Psychodynamic Nursing* (New York: Putnam).

Peplau, H.E. (1988) *Interpersonal Relations in Nursing* (London: Macmillan).

Petrie, P. (1997) *Communicating with Children and Adults: Interpersonal Skills for Early Years and Play Work* (London: Arnold).

Ruesch, J. (1961) *Therapeutic Communication* (Toronto: Norton & Company Inc).

Sheppard, M. (1993) Client satisfaction, extended intervention and interpersonal skills in community mental health, *Journal of Advanced Nursing*, 18: 246–59.

Thorsteinsson, L.S.C.H. (2002) The quality of nursing care as perceived by individuals with chronic illnesses: The magical touch of nursing. *Journal of Clinical Nursing*, 11: 32–44.

Wilkinson, S. (1999) Communication: It makes a difference. *Cancer Nursing*, 22: 17–20.

Chapter 2

Alligood, M.R. (2006a) Philosophies, models, and theories: Critical thinking structures. In Alligood, M.R. and Marriner-Tomey, A. (eds) *Nursing Theory Utilization and Application*, 3rd edn (London: Mosby), pp. 43–66.

Alligood, M.R. (2006b) The nature of knowledge needed for nursing practice. In Alligood, M.R. and Marriner-Tomey, A. (eds)

Nursing Theory Utilization and Application, 3rd edn (London: Mosby), pp. 3–16.

An Bord Altranais (2010) *Guidance for New Nurse and Midwife Registrants* (Dublin: An Bord Altranais).

Arnold, E.C. and Underman Boggs, K. (2011) *Interpersonal Relationships-Professional Communication Skills for Nurses*, 6th edn (St. Louis, MO: Saunders).

Barker, P. (2001) The tidal model: Developing an empowering person centred approach to recovery within psychiatric and mental health nursing. *Journal of Psychiatric and Mental Health Nursing* 8(3): 233–40.

Costa, M.J. (2001) The lived perioperative experience of ambulatory surgery patients. *AORN Journal*, 74(6): 874–81.

Fawcett, J. (2005) *Contemporary Nursing Knowledge: Analysis and Evaluation of Nursing Models and Theories*, 2nd edn (Philadelphia: F.A. Davies Company).

Griffiths, P. (1998) An investigation into the description of patients' problems by nurses using two different needs-based nursing models. *Journal of Advanced Nursing*, 28(5) 969–77.

Health Information and Quality Authority (HIQA) (2010) *Draft National Standards for Safer Better Care Consultation Document* (Dublin: HIQA).

Holland, K. (2008) An introduction to the Roper Logan Tierney Model of care. In Holland, K., Jenkins, J., Solomon, J. and Whittam, S. (eds) *Applying the Roper Logan Tierney Model in Practice*, 2nd edn (London: Churchill Livingstone) pp. 3–22.

Holland, K., Jenkins, J., Solomon, J. and Whittam, S. (eds) (2008) *Applying the Roper Logan Tierney Model in Practice*, 2nd edn (London: Churchill Livingstone).

Iggulden, H. (2008) Communicating. In Holland, K., Jenkins, J., Solomon, J. and Whittam, S. (eds) *Applying the Roper Logan Tierney Model in Practice*, 2nd edn (London: Churchill Livingstone) pp. 101–36.

Jenner, E.A. (1998) A case study analysis of nurses' roles, education and training needs associated with patient-focused care. *Journal of Advanced Nursing*, 27(50): 1087–95.

Kim, H.S. (1983) *The Nature of Theoretical Thinking in Nursing* (Norwalk, CT: Appleton-Century Crofts).

Lee, P. (2003) Children's nursing: Can it justify a separate existence in the UK? *Journal of Advanced Nursing*, 12(5): 762–94.

Martin, G. (1998) Ritual action and its effect on the role of the nurse as advocate. *Journal of Advanced Nursing*, 27(1): 189–94.

Mason, C. (1999) 'Guide to practice' or 'load of rubbish'? The influence of care plans on nursing practice in five clinical areas in Northern Ireland. *Journal of Advanced Nursing*, 29(2): 380–7.

McCabe, C. (2004) Nurse-patient communication: An exploration of patients' experiences. *Journal of Clinical Nursing*, 13(1): 41–9.

McCrae, N. (2012) Whither nursing models? The value of nursing theory in the context of evidence-based practice and multidisciplinary health care. *Journal of Advanced Nursing*, 68(1): 222–9.

Melia, K.M. (1998) Learning and working. The occupational socialisation of nurses. In Mackay, L., Soothill, K. and Melia, K.M. (eds) *Classic Texts in HealthCare* (Oxford: Reed Educational), pp. 154–9.

Murphy, K., Cooney, A., Casey, D., Connor, M. O'Connor, J. and Dineen, B. (2000) The Roper, Logan and Tierney Model: Perceptions and operationalization of the model in psychiatric nursing within one health board in Ireland. *Journal of Advanced Nursing* 31(6): 1333–41.

Notara, V., Koupidis, S.A., Vaga, E. and Grammatikopoulos, I.A. (2010) Economic crisis and challenges for the Greek healthcare system: The emergent role of nursing management. *Journal of Nursing Management* 18(5): 501–4.

Nursing and Midwifery Council (NMC) (2010) *Standards for Pre-registration Nursing Education* (London: Nursing and Midwifery Council).

Orem, D.E. (1971, 1980, 1985, 1991, 1995, 2001) *Nursing: Concepts of Practice*, six editions (London: Mosby).

Paton, B.I. (2009) The professional practice knowledge of nurse preceptors. *Journal of Nursing Education*, 49(3): 143–9.

Pearson, A., Vaughan, B. and Fitzgerald, M. (2005) *Nursing Models for Practice*, 3rd edn (Oxford: Butterworth Heinemann).

Peplau, H.E. (1952, 1991) *Interpersonal Relations in Nursing A Conceptual Frame of Reference for Psychodynamic Nursing* (New York: Springer).

Riley, J.P., Bullock, I., West, S. and Shuldham, C. (2003) Practical application of educational rhetoric: A pathway to expert cardiac nurse practice? *European Journal of Cardiovascular Nursing*, 2(4): 283–90.

Roper, N., Logan, W.W. and Tierney, A. J. (1980, 1985, 1990, 1996) *The Elements of Nursing A Model for Nursing Based on a Model for Living*, four editions (London: Churchill Livingstone).

Roper, N., Logan, W.W. and Tierney, A.J. (2001) *The Roper Logan Tierney Model of Nursing Based on Activities of Living* (London: Churchill Livingstone).

Sims-Williams, A.J. (1976) Temperature taking with glass thermometers: A review. *Journal of Advanced Nursing*, 1, 481–93.

Smith F. (1995) *Children's Nursing in Practice: The Nottingham Model* (Oxford: Blackwell).

Thompson, D. (2002) Nurse-directed services: How can they be made more effective? *European Journal of Cardiovascular Nursing*, 1(1): 7–10.

Thompson, H.J. and Kagan, S.H. (2011) Clinical management of fever by nurses: Doing what works. *Journal of Advanced Nursing*, 67(2): 359–70.

Timmins, F., Mc Cabe, C., Griffiths, C., Gleeson, M. and O'Shea, J. (2005) *Lessons from Practice – Reflection on Communication across the Disciplines*. Royal College of Nursing of the United Kingdom Research Society Annual International Nursing Research Conference 9–11th March, Belfast.

Ward, M. and Jackson, A. (2006) Incorporation of the tidal model into the interdisciplinary plan of care – a program quality improvement project. *Journal of Psychiatric & Mental Health Nursing*, 13(4): 464–7

Wheeler, N.L. (2010) Dementia care 1: person centred approaches help to promote effective communication. *Nursing Times*, 106(24): 18–21.

Wimpenny, P. (2001) The meaning of models of nursing to practicing nurses. *Journal of Advanced Nursing*, 40(3): 346–54

Wissow, L.S. (2004) Communication and malpractice claims – where are we now? *Patient Education and Counseling*, 52(1): 13–15.

Chapter 3

An Bord Altranais (2005) *An Bord Altranais Requirements and Standards for Nurse Registration Education programmes*. (Dublin: An Bord Altranais).

Arnold, E.C. and Underman Boggs, K. (2011) *Interpersonal Relationships – Professional Communication Skills for Nurses*, 6th edn (St. Louis, MO: Saunders).

Buber, M. (1958) *I and Thou*, 2nd edn, R.G. Smith (trans.) (New York: Scribner).

Burnard, P. and Gill, P. (2009) *Culture, Communication and Nursing* (London: Pearson).

Coyle, J. and Williams, B. (2001) Valuing people as individuals: Development of an instrument through a survey of person-centeredness in secondary care. *Journal of Advanced Nursing*, 36(3): 450–9.

DeVito, J.A. (2011) *Essentials of Human Communication*, 7th edn (London: Pearson).

Hindle, S.A. (2006) Psychological factors affecting communication. In Ellis, R.B., Gates, B. and Kenworthy, N. (eds) *Interpersonal Communication in Nursing*, 2nd edn (Edinburgh: Churchill Livingstone), pp. 53–70.

Langwitz, W.A., Eich, P., Kiss, A. and Wossmer, B. (1998) Improving communication skills – a randomized controlled behaviourally-oriented intervention study for residents in internal medicine. *Psychosomatic Medicine*, 60: 268–76.

Maslow, A.H. (1954) *Motivation and Personality* (New York: Harper & Row).

McCabe, C. (2004) Nurse-patient communication: An exploration of patients' experiences. *Journal of Clinical Nursing*, 13: 41–9.

McCormack, B. and McCance, T. (2006) Development of a framework for person-centred nursing. *Journal of Advanced Nursing*, 56(5): 472–9.

Morrissey, J. and Callaghan, P. (2011) *Communication Skills for Mental Health Nurses: An Introduction* (Glasgow: Open University Press/McGraw Hill).

Morse, J.M., De Luca Havens, G.A. and Wilson, S. (1997) The comforting interaction: Developing a model of nurse-patient relationship. *Scholarly Inquiry for Nursing Practice*, 11(4): 321–43.

Peplau, H.E. (1952) *Interpersonal Relations in Nursing* (New York: Putnam).

Rogers, C.R. (1961) *On Becoming a Person* (Boston: Houghton Mifflin).

Suikkala, A., Leino-Kilipi, H. and Katajisto, J. (2009) Factors related to the nursing student-patient relationship: The patient's perspective. *Scandinavian Journal of Caring Sciences*, 23(4): 625–34.

Wheeler, N.L. (2010) Dementia care 1: Person centred approaches help to promote effective communication. *Nursing Times*, 106(24): 18–21.

Chapter 4

Argyle, M., Salter, V., Nicholson, H., Williams, M. and Burgess, P. (1970) The communication of inferior and superior attitudes by verbal and non-verbal signals. *British Journal of Social and Clinical Psychology*, 9: 222–31.

DeVito, J.A. (2011) *Essentials of Human Communication*, 7th edn (London: Pearson).

Fleischer, S., Berg, A., Zimmermann, M., Wuste, K. and Behrens, J. (2009) Nurse-patient interaction and communication: A systematic literature review. *Journal of Public Health*, 17: 339–53.

Freshwater D. (2003) *Counselling Skills for Nurses, Midwives and Health Visitor* (Maidenhead: Open University Press).

Gibbons, M.B. (1993) Listening to the lived experience of loss. *Pediatric Nursing*, 6: 597–9.

Hargie, O. (2011) *Skilled Interpersonal Communication* (London: Routledge).

Kunyk, D. (2001) Clarification of conceptualizations of empathy. *Journal of Advanced Nursing*, 35(3): 317–25.

McCabe, C. (2004) Nurse-patient communication: An exploration of patients' experiences. *Journal of Clinical Nursing*, 13: 41–9.

McCabe, C. (2010) Communication and conflict resolution. In Brady, A.M. (ed.) *Leadership and Management in the Irish Health Service* (Dublin: Gill & Macmillan Ltd).

Morse, J.M., Bottorff, J., Anderson, G., O'Brien, B. and Solberg, S. (1992) Beyond empathy: Expanding expressions of caring. *Journal of Advanced Nursing*, 17: 809–21.

Peplau, H.E. (1997) Peplau's theory of interpersonal relations. *Nursing Science Quarterly*, 10(4): 162–7.

Perry, B. (1996) Influence of nurse gender on the use of silence, touch and humour. *International Journal of Palliative Nursing*, 7: 7–14.

Reynolds, W. and Scott, P.A. (2000) Nursing, empathy and perception of the moral. *Journal of Advanced Nursing*, 32(1): 235–42.

Roberts, L. and Bucksey, S. (2007) Communication with patients: What happens in practice? *Physical Therapy*, 87: 586–94.

Washer, P. (2009) Writing about patients. In Washer, P. (ed.) *Clinical Communication Skills* (New York: Oxford University Press), pp. 38–43.

Williams, A. (2001) A study of practicing nurses' perceptions and experiences of intimacy within the nurse-patient relationship. *Journal of Advanced Nursing*, 32(2): 188–96.

Wiseman T. (1996) A concept analysis of empathy. *Journal of Advanced Nursing*, 23(6): 1162–7.

Chapter 5

Aggleton, P. and Chalmers, H. (2000) *Nursing Models and Nursing Practice*, 2nd edn (Basingstoke: Palgrave).

An Bord Altranais (2010) *Guidance for New Nurse and Midwife Registrants* (Dublin: An Bord Altranais).

Arnold, E.C. and Underman Boggs, K. (2011) *Interpersonal Relationships-Professional Communication Skills for Nurses*, 6th edn (St. Louis, MO: Saunders).

Betts, A. (2001) Improving communication. In Ellis, R.B., Gates, R.J. and Kenworthy, N. (eds) *Interpersonal Communication in Nursing Theory and Practice*, 2nd edn (London: Churchill Livingstone), pp. 73–83.

Bowler, I.M.W. (1993) Stereotypes of women of Asian descent in midwifery: Some evidence. *Midwifery*, 9(1): 7–16.

Burnard, P. (1997) *Effective Communication Skills for Health Professionals*, 2nd edn (Cheltenham: Nelson Thornes).

Burnard, P. and Gill, P. (2008) *Culture, Communication and Nursing* (Edinburgh: Pearson).

Chambers-Evans, J., Stelling, J. and Godin, M. (1999) Learning to listen: Serendipitous outcomes of a research training experience. *Journal of Advanced Nursing* 29(6): 1421–6.

Corbett, T. (2001) The nurse as a professional carer. In Ellis, R.B., Gates, R.J., Kenworthy, N. (eds) *Interpersonal Communication in Nursing Theory and Practice* (London: Churchill Livingstone 2001), pp. 91–107.

Costa, M.J. (2001) The lived perioperative experience of ambulatory surgery patients. *AORN Journal*, 74(6): 874–81.

Coyle, J. and Williams, B. (2001) Valuing people as individuals: Development of an instrument through a survey of person-centeredness in secondary care. *Journal of Advanced Nursing*, 36(3): 450–59.

Cree, V.E., Kay, H., Tisdall, K., and Wallace, J. (2004) Stigma and parental HIV. *Qualitative Social Work* 3(1): 7–25.

Davies, M.M. and Bath, P.A. (2001) The maternity information concerns of Somali women in the United Kingdom. *Journal of Advanced Nursing*, 36(2): 237–45.

DeVito, J.A. (2009) *Human Communication – The Basic Course*, 12th edn (London: Pearson).

DeVito, J.A. (2011) *Essentials of Human Communication*, 7th edn (London: Pearson).

Doak, C.C., Doak, L.G. and Root, J.H. (1985) *Teaching Patients with Low Literacy Skill* (Philadelphia: J.B. Lippincott).

Driscoll, A. (2000) Managing post-discharge care at home: An analysis of patients' and their carers' perceptions of information received during their stay in hospital. *Journal of Advanced Nursing*, 31(5): 1165–73.

Edwards, S.C. (1998) An anthropological interpretation of nurses' and patients' perceptions of the use of space and touch. *Journal of Advanced Nursing*, 28(4): 809–17.

Edwards, A., Evans, R. and Elwyn, G. (2003) Manufactured but not imported: New directions for research in shared decision making support and skills. *Patient Education and Counseling*, 50(1): 33–8.

Fallowfield, L., Jenkins, V., Farewell, V., Saul, J., Duffy, A., and Eves, R. (2002) Efficacy of a cancer research UK communication skills training model for oncologists: A randomised controlled trial. *Lancet*, 359 (Feb. 22): 650–6.

Fossum, B. and Arborelius, E. (2004) Patient-centred communication: Videotaped consultations. *Patient Education and Counseling*, 54: 163–9.

Foster, J.H. and Onyeukwu, C. (2003) The attitudes of forensic nurses to substance using service users. *Journal of Psychiatric and Mental Health Nursing*, 10(5): 578–84.

Gallant, M.H., Beaulieu, M.C. and Carnveale, F.A. (2002) Partnership: An analysis of the concept within the nurse-client relationship. *Journal of Advanced Nursing*, 40(2): 149–57.

Gibbons, M.B. (1993) Listening to the lived experience of loss. *Pediatric Nursing*, 6: 597–9.

Hargie, O. (2011) *Skilled Interpersonal Communication* (London: Routledge).

Hindle, S.A. (2006) Pyschological factors affecting communication. In Ellis, R.B., Gates, B. and Kenworthy, N. (eds) *Interpersonal Communication in Nursing*, 2nd edn (Edinburgh: Churchill Livingstone), pp. 53–70.

Ito, M. and Lambert, V.A. (2002) Communication effectiveness of nurses working in a variety of settings within one large university teaching hospital in western Japan. *Nursing and Health Sciences*, 4: 149–53.

Jarrett N.J. and Payne S.A. (2000) Creating and maintaining 'optimism' in cancer care communication. *International Journal of Nursing Studies*, 37: 81–90.

Jorm, A.F., Korten, A.E., Jacomb, P.A., Christensen, H. and Henderson, S. (1999) Attitudes toward people with a mental disorder: A survey of the Australian public and health professionals. *Australian and New Zealand Journal of Psychiatry*, 33: 77–83.

Kalb, K.B., Cherry, N.M., Kauzloric, J., Brender, A., Green, K., Miyagawa, L. and Shinoda-Mettler, A. (2006) A competency-based approach. *Public Health Nursing* 23(2): 115–38.

Keating, D., Bellchambers, H., Bujack, E., Cholowski, K., Conway, J. and Neal, P. (2002) Communication: Principal barrier to nurse-consumer partnerships. *International Journal of Nursing Practice*, 8: 16–22.

Kirkham, M., Stapleton, H., Curtis, P. and Thomas, G. (2002) Stereotyping as a professional defence mechanism. *British Journal of Midwifery*, 10(9): 549–52.

Mavundla, T.R. and Uys, LR. (1997) The attitudes of nurses toward mentally ill people in a general hospital setting in Durban. *Curationis*, 20(2): 3–7.

McCabe, C. (2004) Nurse-patient communication: An exploration of patients' experiences. *Journal of Clinical Nursing*, 13: 41–9.

Michie, S., Miles, J. and Weinman, J. (2003) Patient-centredness in chronic illness: What is it and does it matter? *Patient Education and Counseling*, 51: 197–260.

Miller, G.R. and Nicholson, H.E. (1976) *Communication Inquiry: A Perspective on Process* (Reading: Addison-Wesley).

Morrall, P. (2003) Social factors affecting communication. In Ellis, R.B., Gates, R.J., and Kenworthy, N. (eds) *Interpersonal Communication in Nursing Theory and Practice*, 2nd edn (London: Churchill Livingstone), pp. 33–51.

Nursing and Midwifery Council (NMC) (2010) *Standards for Pre-registration Nursing Education* (London: Nursing and Midwifery Council).

O'Brien, L. (2000) Nurse–client relationships: The experience of community psychiatric nurses. *Australian and New Zealand Journal of Mental Health Nursing*, 9(4): 184–94.

Orem, D.E. (2001) *Nursing: Concepts of Practice*, 6th edn (London: Mosby).

Pearson, A., Vaughan, B. and Fitzgerald, M. (2005) *Nursing Models for Practice*, 3rd edn (Oxford: Butterworth Heinemann).

Peplau, H.E. (1952, 1991) *Interpersonal Relations in Nursing A Conceptual Frame of Reference for Psychodynamic Nursing* (New York: Springer).

Röndahl, G., Innala, S. and Carlsson, M. (2004) Nurses' attitudes towards lesbians and gay men. *Journal of Advanced Nursing*, 47:386–92.

Roper, N., Logan, W.W. and Tierney, A.J. (2001) *The Roper Logan Tierney Model of Nursing Based on Activities of Living* (London: Churchill Livingstone).

Sidell, M. (2000) Supporting individuals and facilitating change: The role of counselling skills. In Katz, J., Perberdy, A. and Douglas, J. (eds) *Promoting Health: Knowledge and Practice* (London: Palgrave), pp. 140–61.

Simons, J. and Robertson, E. (2002) Poor communication and knowledge deficits: Obstacles to effective management of children's postoperative pain. *Journal of Advanced Nursing*, 40(1): 78–86.

Suikkala, A., Leino-Kilipi, H. and Katajisto, J. (2009) Factors related to the nursing student-patient relationship: The patient's perspective. *Scandinavian Journal of Caring Sciences*, 23(4): 625–34.

Tierney, A.J. (1998) Nursing models extant or extinct? *Journal of Advanced Nursing*, 8(1): 77–85.

Uitterhoeve, R., De Leeuw, J., Bensing, J., Heaven, C., Borm, G., Demulder, P. and Van Achterberg, T. (2008) Cue-responding behaviours of oncology nurses in video-simulated interviews. *Journal of Advanced Nursing*, 61: 71–80.

Wheeler, N.L. (2010) Dementia care 1: Person centred approaches help to promote effective communication. *Nursing Times*, 106(24): 18–21.

Wilkinson, S., Linsell, I., Perry, R. and Blanchard, K. (2008a) Communication skills training for nurses working with patients with heart disease. *British Journal of Cardiac Nursing*, 3(10): 475–81.

Wilkinson, S., Perry, R., Blanchard, K., and Linsell, L. (2008b) Effectiveness of a three-day communication skills course in changing nurses' communication skills with cancer/palliative care patients: A randomised controlled trial. *Palliative Medicine* 12: 365–75.

Williams, K., Kemper, S. and Hummert, L. (2004) Enhancing communication with older adults: Overcoming elderspeak. *Journal of Gerontological Nursing*, 30(10): 17–25.

Zion, A.B. and Aiman, J. (1989) Level of reading difficulty in American College of Obstetrics and Gynaecology patient education pamphlets. *Obstetrics and Gynaecology*, 74, 6: 955–60.

Chapter 6

Alberti, R.E. and Emmons, M.E. (1986) *Your Perfect Right: A Guide to Assertive Behaviour*, 4th edn (St. Lois Obispo, CA: Impact)

Arnold, E.C. and Underman Boggs, K. (2011) *Interpersonal Relationships-Professional Communication Skills for Nurses*, 6th edn (St. Louis, MO: Saunders).

Balzer-Riley, J. (2011) *Communication in Nursing*, 7th edn (St. Louis, MO: Mosby).

Brechin, A., Brown, H. and Eby, M. (2000) (eds) *Critical Practice in Health and Social Care* (London: Sage).

Brinkett, R. (2010) A literature review of conflict communication causes, costs, benefits and interventions in nursing. *Journal of Nursing Management*, 18, 145–56.

DeVito, J.A. (2011) *Essentials of Human Communication*, 7th edn (London: Pearson).

Dowling, S., Martin, R., Skidmore, P., Doyal, L., Cameron, A. and Lloyd, S. (2000) Nurses taking on junior doctors work: A confusion of accountability. In Davies, C., Finlay, L. and Bullman, A. (eds) *Changing Practice in Health and Social Care* (London, Sage Publications), pp. 326–34.

Hargie, O. (2011) *Skilled Interpersonal Communication* (Routledge, London).

McCabe, C. and Timmins, F. (2003) Teaching assertiveness to undergraduate nursing students. *Nurse Education in Practice* 3(1): 30–42.

McCartan, P. (2001) The identification and analysis of assertive behaviours in nurses. University of Ulster: School of Nursing and Midwifery, unpublished PhD thesis.

Milstead, J.A. (1996) Basic tools for the orthopaedic staff nurse–part II: Conflict management and negotiation. *Orthopaedic Nursing* 15(2): 39–45.

Percival, J. (2001) Don't be too nice *Nursing Standard*, 15(19): 22.

Poroch, D. and McIntosh, W. (1995) Barriers to assertive skills in nurses. *Australian and New Zealand Journal of Mental Health Nursing*, 4: 113–23.

Rosenblatt, C.L. and Davis, M.S. (2009) Effective communication techniques for managers. *Nursing Management*, 40(6): 52–4.

Taylor, B. (1989) *Assertiveness and the Management of Conflict: Including Supplementary Trainer's Workshop Notes* (Leeds: Beechwood Conference Centre).

Thompson, N. (2009) *People Skills*, 3rd edn (Basingstoke: Palgrave Macmillan).

Timmins, F. and McCabe, C. (2005) Nurses' and midwives' assertive behaviour in the workplace. *Journal of Advanced Nursing*, 51(1): 38-45.

Valentine, P.E.B. (1995) Management of conflict: do nurses/women handle it differently? *Journal of Advanced Nursing*, 22: 142–9.

Willis, L. and Daisley, J. (1994) *Springboard Women's Developmental Workbook* (Stroud: Hawthorne Press).

Willis, L. and Daisley, J. (1995) *The Assertive Trainer A Practical Handbook for Trainers and Running Assertiveness Courses* (Maidenhead: McGraw-Hill).

Chapter 7

Beckett, C.D. and Kipnis, G. (2009) Collaborative communication: Integrating SBAR to improve quality/patient safety outcomes. *Journal for Healthcare Quality*, 31(5): 19–29.

DeVito, J.A. (2011) *Essentials of Human Communication*, 7th edn (London: Pearson).

Dingley, C., Daugherty, K., Derieg, M.K. and Persing, R. (2008) Improving patient safety through provider communication strategy enhancements. In Henriksen, K., Battles, J.B., Keyes, M.A., Grady, M.L. (eds) *Advances in Patient Safety: New Directions and Alternative Approaches*, vol. 3 (Rockville, MD: Agency for Healthcare Research and Quality (US)). Accessed 4 March 2013 at: http://www.ncbi.nlm.nih.gov/books/ NBK43663/

Fewster-Thuente, L. and Velsor-Friedrich, B. (2008) Interdisciplinary collaboration for healthcare professionals. *Nursing Administration Quarterly*, 32(1): 40–8.

Francis, R. (2010) *Independent Inquiry into Care Provided by Mid Staffordshire NHS Foundation Trust January 2005–March 2009 Volume I*. Accessed 4 March 2013 at:http://www.dh.gov.uk/en/ Publicationsandstatistics/Publications/PublicationsPolicyAnd Guidance/DH_113018

Gardner, D. (2005) Ten lessons in collaboration. *OJIN: The Online Journal of Issues in Nursing*. 10(1): ms 1.

Hargie, O. (2011) *Skilled Interpersonal Communication* (Routledge, London).

McCabe, C. (2010) Communication and conflict resolution. In Brady, A.M. (ed) *Leadership & Management in the Irish Health Service* (Dublin: Gill & Macmillan).

Nadzam, D. (2009) Nurses' role in communication and patient safety. *Journal of Nursing Care Quarterly*, 24(3): 184–8.

Orchard, C.A. (2010) Persistent isolationist or collaborator? The nurse's role in interprofessional collaborative practice. *Journal of Nursing Management*, 18: 248–57.

Permanente, K. (2005) *SBAR Technique for Communication: A Situational Briefing Model*. (Cambridge, MA: Institute for Healthcare Improvement). Accessed 4 March 2013 at: http:// www.ihi.org/knowledge/pages/tools/sbartechniquefor communicationasituationalbriefingmodel.aspx

Rains, S.A. and Turner, M. (2007) Psychological reactance and persuasive health communication: A test and extension of the intertwined model. *Human Communication Research*, 22: 241–69.

Reber, P.A., DiPietro, E.A., Paraway, Y., Obst, B.P., Smith, R.A. and Koller, C.L. (2011) Communication: The key to effective interdisciplinary collaboration in the care of a child with complex rehabilitation needs. *Rehabilitation Nursing*, 36(5): 181–5.

Reeves, S. (2009) An overview of continuing interprofessional education. *Journal of Continuing Education in the Health Professions*, 29(3): 142–6.

Sahlsten, M.J., Larsson, I.E., Sjostrom, B., Lindencrona, C. and Plos, K. (2007) Patient participation in nursing care: Towards a concept clarification from a nurse perspective. *Journal of Clinical Nursing*, 16: 630–7.

Thompson, J.E., Collett, L.W., Langbart, M.J., Purcell, N.J., Boyd, S.M., Yuminaga, Y., Ossolinski, G., Susanto, C. and McCormack, A. (2011) Using the ISBAR handover tool in junior medical officer handover: A study in an Australian tertiary hospital. *Postgrad Medical Journal* 87: 340–4.

Wright, D. and Brajtman, S. (2011) Relational and embodied knowing: Nursing ethics within the interprofessional team. *Nursing Ethics*, 18 (1): 20–30.

Chapter 8

Anon. (1994) Cot death – A mother's story. *New World of Irish Nursing*, 2(1): 10–12.

Craib I. (1999) Reflections on mourning in the modern world. *International Journal of Palliative Nursing*, 5(2): 87–9.

Engel, G.L. (1972) Grief and grieving. In L. Schwartz and S. Schwartz (eds) *The Psychodynamics of Patient Care* (New York: Prentice Hall), pp. 376–87.

Giger, J.N. and Davidhizar, R.E. (1999) *Transcultural Nursing: Assessment & Intervention*, 3rd edn (St. Louis, MO: Mosby).

Grypma S. (1993) Culture shock. *The Canadian Nurse*, Sept.: 33–6.

Harms, L. (2007) *Working with People: Communication Skills for Reflective Practice* (Victoria: Oxford University Press).

Jones D.C. and Van Amelsvoort-Jones, G.M.M. (1986) Communication patterns between nursing staff and the ethnic elderly in a long-term care facility. *Journal of Advanced Nursing*, 11(3): 265–72.

Kreigh H. and Perko J. (1983) *Psychiatric and Mental Health Nursing: A Commitment to Care and Concern*, 2nd edn (Reston VA: Reston Publishing Company).

Kubler-Ross, E. (1973) *On Death and Dying* (London: Tavistock).

Lea, A. (1994) Nursing in today's multicultural society: A transcultural perspective. *Journal of Advanced Nursing*, 20: 307–13.

Leininger, M. (1991) Transcultural nursing: The study and practice field. *Imprint*, 38(2): 55–66.

Lindemann, E. (1944) Symptomatology and management of acute grief. *American Journal of Psychiatry*, 101: 141–8.

Moser, D., Chung, M., McKinley, S., Riegel, B., An, K., Cherrington, C., Blakely, W., Biddle, M., Frazier, S. and Garvin, B. (2003) Critical care nursing practice regarding patient anxiety assessment and management. *Intensive and Critical Care Nursing*, 19(5): 276–88.

Stockwell, F. (1972) *The Unpopular Patient* (London: Royal College of Nursing).

Windsor-Richards, K. and Gillies, P.A. (1988) Racial grouping and women's experiences of giving birth in hospital. *Midwifery*, 4: 171–6.

Wollett, A. and Dosanjh-Matwala, N. (1990) Pregnancy and Antenatal Care: the attitudes and experiences of Asian women, in *Child: Care, Health and Development*, Jan–Feb, 16(1): 63–78.

Chapter 9

Basford, L. and Slevin, O. (2003) *Theory and Practice of Nursing: An Integrated Approach to Caring Practice*, 2nd edn (Cheltenham: Nelson Thornes).

Bateman, N. (2000) *Advocacy Skills for Health and Social Care Professionals* (London: Jessica Kingsley Publishers).

Bowker, G.C., Star, S. and Spasser, M. (2001) Classifying nursing work. *Online Journal of Issues in Nursing* 6(2, March). Accessed 4 March 2013 at: www.nursingworld.org/MainMenuCategories/ANAMarketplace/ANAPeriodicals/OJIN/TableofContents/Volume62001/No2May01/ArticlePreviousTopic/ClassifyingNursingWork.aspx

Clark, J. and Lang, N. (1992) Nursing's next advance: An international classification for nursing practice. *International Journal of Nursing* 39(4): 102–12.

Colyer, H.M. (2004) The construction and development of health professions: Where will it end? *Journal of Advanced Nursing*, 48(4): 406–12.

Dimond, B. (1999) *Patients' Rights, Responsibilities and the Nurse*, 2nd edn (Dinton, UK: Quay Books).

Gates, B. (1994) *Advocacy: A Nurses' Guide* (London: Scutari Press).

Gaudine, A., LeFort, S.M., Lamb, M. and Thorne, L. (2011) Clinical ethical conflicts of nurses and physicians. *Nursing Ethics*, 18(1): 9–19.

Hancock, H. (1997) Professional responsibility: Implications for nursing practice within the realms of cardiothoracics. *Journal of Advanced Nursing*, 25: 1054–60.

Hanks, R.G. (2010) The medical-surgical nurse perspective of advocate role. *Nursing Forum*, 45(2): 97–107.

Hart, C. (2004) *Nurses and Politics; The Impact of Power and Practice* (London: Palgrave Macmillan).

Henderson, V. (1966) *The Nature of Nursing: A Definition and its Implications for Practice, Research, and Education* (New York: Macmillan).

Liaschenko, J. and Peter, E. (2004) Nursing ethics and conceptualisations of nursing: Profession, practice and work. *Journal of Advanced Nursing*, 46(5): 488–95.

Llewellyn, P. (2004) Nursing and advocacy in person-centred planning. *Learning Disability Practice*, 7(9): 14–17.

Mason, D.L. (2011) The nursing profession: Development, challenges and opportunities. In Mason, D.L., Isaacs, S.L. and Colby, D.C. (eds) *The Nursing Profession: Development, Challenges and Opportunities* (San Francisco: Jossey-Bass), pp. 3–82.

McCabe, C. and Timmins, F. (2012) *Communicating care*. In McSherry, W., McSherry, R. and Watson, R. (eds) *Care In Nursing: Principles, Values, and Skills* (Oxford: Oxford University Press), pp. 137–49.

McDonald, H. (2007) Relational ethics and advocacy in nursing: Literature review. *Journal of Advanced Nursing*, 57(2): 119–26.

McSherry, R. and Pearce, P. (2011) *Clinical Governance: A Guide to Implementation for Healthcare Professions* (Oxford: Wiley Blackwell).

Milton, C.L. (2008) Accountability in nursing; Reflecting on ethical codes and professional standards of nursing practice from a global perspective. *Nursing Science Quarterly*, 21(4): 300–3.

Negarandeh, R., Oskouie, F., Ahmadi, F., Nikravesh, M. and Hallberg, I.R. (2006) Patient advocacy: Barriers and facilitators. *BMC Nursing*, 5:3.

Oxford English Dictionary (2012) Advocate (Oxford: Oxford University Press).

Peter, E., Lunardi, V.L. and Macfarlane, A. (2004) Nursing resistance as ethical action: Literature review. *Journal of Advanced Nursing*, 46(4): 403–16.

Redman, B.K. and Fry, S.T. (2000) Nurses' ethical conflicts: What is really about them? *Nursing Ethics*, 7(4): 360–6.

Reed, P. (2011) The ontology of the discipline. In Cody, W. (ed.) *Philosophical and Theoretical Perspectives for Advancing Nursing Practice* (Burlington MA: Jones & Bartlett Learning), pp. 73–9.

Rich, K. (2007) Introduction to ethical philosophy, theories and approaches. In Butts, J. and Rich, K. (eds) *Nursing Ethics: Across the Curriculum and Into Practice* (London, Jones & Bartlett Publishers), pp. 39–80.

Rogers, C.R. (1961) *On Becoming a Person* (Boston, MA: Houghton Mifflin).

Rutherford, M. (2008) Standardized nursing language: What does it mean for nursing practice? *OJIN: The Online Journal of Issues in Nursing*, 13(1). Accessed 4 March 2013 at: http://www.nursing-world.org/MainMenuCategories/ThePracticeofProfessional Nursing/Health-IT/StandardizedNursingLanguage.html

Rutty, J.E. (1998) The nature of philosophy of science, theory and knowledge relating to nursing and professionalism. *Journal of Advanced Nursing*, 28(2): 243–50.

Shaw, H.K. and Degazon, C. (2008) Integrating the core professional values of nursing: A profession, not just a career. *Journal of Cultural Diversity*, 15(1): 44–50.

Takase, M., Kershaw, E. and Burt, L. (2001) Nurse-environment misfit and nursing practice. *Journal of Advanced Nursing*, 35(6): 819–26.

Tschudin, V. (2003) *Ethics in Nursing: The Caring Relationship*, 3rd edn (London: Butterworth Heinemann).

Vaartio, H., Leino-Kilpi, H., Suommen, T. and Pukka, P. (2008) The content of advocacy in procedural pain care – patients and nurses' perspectives, *Journal of Advanced Nursing*, 64(5): 504–13.

Chapter 10

Arnold, E.C. and Underman Boggs, K. (2011) *Interpersonal Relationships – Professional Communication Skills for Nurses*, 6th edn (St Louis, MO: Saunders).

Bandura, A. (1977) Self-efficacy: Toward a unifying theory of behavioral change. *Psychological Review*, 84(2): 191–215.

Bandura, A. (1986) *Social Foundations of Thought and Action: A Social Cognitive Theory* (Englewood Cliffs, NJ: Prentice Hall).

Bandura, A. (1997) *Self-Efficacy: The Exercise of Control* (New York: Freeman).

Barnett, R. (1997) *Higher Education: A Critical Business* (Buckingham: SRHE and Open University Press).

Betts, A. (2003) Improving communication. In Ellis, R.B., Gates, B. and Kenworthy, N. (eds) *Interpersonal Communication in Nursing*

Theory and Practice, 2nd edn (London: Churchill Livingstone), pp. 73–83.

Brechin, A., Brown, H. and Eby, M. (2000) (eds) *Critical Practice in Health and Social Care* (London, Sage).

Bulman, C. and Schutz, S. (2008) *Reflective Practice in Nursing: The Growth of the Professional Practitioner*, 4th edn (Oxford, Blackwell).

Burnard, P. (1985) *Learning Human Skills* (London: Heinemann).

Burnard, P. (1997) *Know Yourself! Self-Awareness Activities for Nurses and Other Health Professionals*, 2nd edn (London: Whurr Publishers Limited).

Carroll, M., Curtis, L., Higgins, A., Nicholl, H., Redmond, R. and Timmins, F. (2002) Is there a place for reflective practice in the nursing curriculum? *Clinical Effectiveness in Nursing*, 6(1): 36-41.

Davidhizar, R. (1993) Self-confidence: A requirement for collaborative practice. *Dimensions of Critical Care Nursing*, 12: 218–22.

Department of Health (2012) Review of undergraduate nursing and midwifery programmes. Dublin: The Department of Health. Accessed 5 March 2013 at: http://www.dohc.ie/publications/pdf/nmr_review_may.pdf?direct=1 accessed

DeVito, J.A. (2011) *Essentials of Human Communication*, 7th edn (London: Pearson).

Dewey, J. (1933) *How We Think* (Boston, MA: Heath & Co.).

Ellis, R.B., Gates, B. and Kenworthy, N. (eds) (2003) *Interpersonal Communication in Nursing Theory and Practice*, 2nd edn (London: Churchill Livingstone), pp. 73–83.

Gibbs, G. (1988) *Learning by Doing: A Guide to Teaching Learning Methods* (Oxford: Oxford Brookes University).

Hannigan, B. (2001) A discussion of the strengths and weaknesses of 'reflection' in nursing practice and education. *Journal of Clinical Nursing*, 10(2): 278–83.

Jensen, S.K. and Joy, C. (2005) Exploring a model to evaluate levels of reflection in baccalaureate nursing student's journals. *Journal of Nursing Education*, 44(3): 139–44.

Johns, C. (1996) Visualizing and realizing caring in practice through guided reflection. *Journal of Advanced Nursing*, 24(6): 1135–43.

Johns, C. (2002) *Guided Reflection: Advancing Practice* (Oxford: Blackwell).

Johns, C. (2009) *Becoming a Reflective Practitioner* (London: Wiley).

Kantcheva, D.A. and Eckroth-Bucher, M. (2002) Self-awareness in psychiatric nursing. Philosophical basis and practice of self-awareness in psychiatric nursing. *Journal of Psychosocial Nursing and Mental Health Services* 39(2): 32–9.

Luft, J. (1984) *Group Process: An Introduction to Group Dynamics*, 3rd edn (New York: McGraw Hill).

McCabe, C. (2004) Nurse-patient communication: An exploration of patients' experiences. *Journal of Clinical Nursing*, 13: 41–9.

Morse, J.M., De Luca Havens, G.A. and Wilson, S. (1997) The comforting interaction: Developing a model of nurse-patient relationship. *Scholarly Inquiry for Nursing Practice*, 11(4): 321–43.

Nash, C. (2000) Applying reflective practice. In Davies, C., Finlay, L. and Bullman, A. (eds) *Changing Practice in Health and Social Care* (London: Sage).

Newell, R. (2002) Is there a place for reflection in the nursing curriculum? *Clinical Effectiveness in Nursing*, 6(1): 42–3.

NHS Leadership Centre (2004) *Leadership Qualities Framework-a Good Practice Guide* (Warwick: NHS Institute for Innovation and Improvement).

Orem, D.E. (2001) *Nursing: Concepts of Practice*, 6th edn (London: Mosby).

O'Shea, J. (2004) Parents' experiences of the neonatal intensive care unit, 5th Annual Research Conference, 3–5 November 2004. School of Nursing and Midwifery, University of Dublin, Trinity College.

Oxford English Dictionary (2012) Self-awareness. Accessed 5 March at: http://oxforddictionaries.com/definition/self-awareness?q= self-awareness

Pearson, A., Vaughan, B. and Fitzgerald, M. (2005) *Nursing Models for Practice*, 3rd edn (Oxford: Butterworth Heinemann).

Peplau, H.E. (1991) *Interpersonal Relations in Nursing: A Conceptual Frame of Reference for Psychodynamic Nursing* (New York: Springer).

Pinkery, S. (2000) Anti-oppressive theory and practice in social work. In Davies, C., Finlay, L. and Bullman, A. (eds) *Changing Practice in Health and Social Care* (London, Sage).

Queendom.com (2012) Tests, tests, tests. Accessed 5 March 2013 at: http://www.queendom.com/tests/ index.html

Rogers, C.R. (1961) *On Becoming a Person* (Boston, MA: Houghton Mifflin).

Rowe, J. (1999) Self-awareness: Improving nurse-client interactions. *Nursing Standard*, 14(8): 37–41.

Scholz, U., Gutiérrez-Doña, B., Sud, S. and Schwarzer, R. (2002) Is perceived self-efficacy a universal construct? Psychometric findings from 25 countries. *European Journal of Psychological Assessment*, 18(3): 242–51.

Schwarzer, R. and Schmitz, G.S. (2004) Perceived self-efficacy and teacher burnout: A Longitudinal Study in ten schools. Presented at the 3rd International Biennial SELF Research Conference Self-Concept , Motivation and Identity: Where to from here? Accessed 24th November 2005 at: http://self.uws.edu.au/ Conferences/2004_Schwarzer_Schmitz.pdf. Abstract accessed 10 March 2013 at: http://trove.nla.gov.au/work/153087608? versionId=166840269

Schön, D. (1983) *The Reflective Practitioner: How Professionals Think in Action* (London: Temple Smith).

Seager, W. (2012) Encyclopedia of consciousness: Philosophical accounts of self-awareness and introspection. Accessed 30 June 2012 at: http:// www.credoreference.com.libezproxy.open.ac.uk/ entry/estcon/philosophical_accounts_of_self_awareness_and_ introspection

Stanford Encyclopedia of Philosophy (2012) *Consciousness*. Accessed 5 March 2013 at: http:// plato.stanford.edu/entries/ consciousness/

Timmins, F. and Dunne, P. (2009) An exploration of the current use and benefit of nursing student portfolios. *Nurse Education Today*, 29: 330–41.

Timmins, F., McCabe, C., Griffiths, C., Gleeson, M., and O'Shea, J. (2005) Lessons from practice – reflection on communication across the disciplines. Symposium Presentation Royal College of Nursing of the United Kingdom Research Society Annual International Nursing Research Conference – 11 March 2005, UK.

Chapter 11

Barnett, R. (1997) *Higher Education: A Critical Business* (Buckingham: SRHE and Open University Press).

Benner, P. (2000) *From Novice to Expert: Excellence and Power in Clinical Nursing Practice* (London Prentice Hall).

Benner, P., Hooper-Kyriakidis, P. and Stannard, D. (1999) *Clinical Wisdom and Interventions in Critical care. A Thinking in Action Approach* (London: W.B. Saunders).

Brechin, A., Brown, H. and Eby. M. (eds) (2000) *Critical Practice in Health and Social Care* (London: Sage).

Fosbinder, D. (1994) Patient perceptions of nursing care: An emerging theory of interpersonal competence. *Journal of Advanced Nursing*, 20: 1085–93.

Gibbs, G. (1988) *Learning by Doing: A Guide to Teaching Learning Methods* (Oxford: Oxford Brookes University).

Gibbs, G., Palmer, A., Burns, S. and Bulman, C. (2000) *Reflective Practice in Nursing* (Oxford: Blackwell).

Jones, L. (2000a) 'Promoting health: everybody's business? In Katz, J., Perberdy, A. and Douglas, J. (eds) *Promoting Health: Knowledge and Practice* (London: Palgrave), pp. 2–17.

Jones, L. (2000b) What is health. In Katz, J., Perberdy, A. and Douglas, J. (eds) *Promoting Health: Knowledge and Practice* (London: Palgrave), pp. 18–36.

Kruijver, J.P.M., Kerkstra, A., Bensing, J.M. and Van de Wiel, H.B.M. (2001) Communication skills of nurses during interactions with simulated cancer patients. *Journal of Advanced Nursing*, 34(6): 772–9.

McCabe, C. (2004) Nurse-patient communication: An exploration of patients' experiences. *Journal of Clinical Nursing*, 13: 41–9.

Morse, J., Bottorff, J., Anderson, G., O'Brien, B. and Solberg, S. (1992) Beyond empathy: Expanding expressions of caring. *Journal of Advanced Nursing*, 17: 809–21.

Morse, J.M., De Luca Havens, G.A. and Wilson, S. (1997) The comforting interaction: Developing a model of nurse-patient relationship. *Scholarly Inquiry for Nursing Practice*, 11(4): 321–43.

O'Donovan, M. (2006) Reflecting during clinical placement – Discovering factors that influence pre-registration psychiatric nursing students. *Nurse Education in Practice* 6(3): 134–40.

Rolfe, G., Freshwater, D. and Jasper, M. (2011) *Critical Reflection in Practice: Generating Knowledge for Care* (Basingstoke: Palgrave Macmillan).

Scholes, J., Webb, C., Gray, M., Endacott, R., Miller, C., Jasper, M. and McMullan, M. (2004) Making portfolios work in practice. *Journal of Advanced Nursing*, 46(6): 595–603.

Sidell, M. (2000) Supporting individuals and facilitating change: The role of counselling skills. In Katz, J., Perberdy, A. and Douglas, J. (eds) *Promoting Health: Knowledge and Practice* (London: Palgrave), pp. 140–61.

Watson, J. (1999) *Post-Modern Nursing and Beyond* (London: Churchill Livingstone).

Watson, J. (n.d.) *Watson's Caring Science*. Accessed 10 March 2013 at: http://watsoncaringscience.org/about-us/caring-science-definitions-processes-theory/

Index

Note: Page numbers in *italics* refer to figures and tables.

Printed and bound by CPI Group (UK) Ltd, Croydon, CR0 4YY